Polly's Principles

Polly's Principles

Polly Bergen tells you how
you can FEEL and LOOK as
YOUNG as she does

BY POLLY BERGEN

Peter H. Wyden/Publisher

NEW YORK

Third Printing, August 1974

LIBRARY OF CONGRESS CATALOG CARD NUMBER: 74-76236

MANUFACTURED IN THE UNITED STATES OF AMERICA

ISBN: 0-88326-073-5

Acknowledgments

Many, many people helped with this book. But I'd like to mention in particular Vernon Scott and the immensely skilled literary collaboration of Kathrin Perutz. Also the professional counsel of George Semel, M.D., Alfred Lerner, M.D., and Max Wolfe, M.D.

P.B.

Contents

Illustrations fall between pages 8-9, 56-57, 88-89, 136-137.

Polly's Principles

1

To Tell The Truth

To Tell The Truth, as you surely know unless you have been living in Tibet, is a very popular TV panel show. I was one of its original panelists and served as its resident philosopher for five years. We didn't always tell the *whole* truth on *To Tell The Truth,* but the show was a lot of laughs, and I think I'm entitled to steal its title to start this book. The words are just right for what I have in mind for you. Which is: to tell the truth about ourselves as women, who we women are, who we want to be, how we get there, and what "Polly's Principles" are—how I acquired them, for what reasons, and what they can do for you. And so I'll start right now by telling the truth about myself, and the best place to start is at the beginning. I guess.

You'll find here what I do about my dieting and my dating, my exercise plan and my sex life, and everything else that makes me look—so people keep telling me—younger than my forty-three years. But mostly I've tried hard to tell you about the key to myself: the way I've come to *feel* about myself. And the way you can come to feel about yourself as well.

I hear some of you saying right now, "OK, but what can a woman like Polly Bergen tell *me,* with *my* problems? What do I have in common with a show-business personality and successful business executive who gets around in places that I only read about and meets people who are only names to me in the newspapers and magazines?"

My suggestion to you is: Read on. My problems have been my own: an unconventional childhood, two failed marriages, one unsuccessful psychoanalysis, and another one that's still going on. But people are people and problems are problems, and overcoming problems—the making of the inner and outer you and me—is universal. And, in some ways, perhaps more difficult to deal with for someone like myself than it might be for you.

Let's see.

Most women assume I was delivered from my mother's womb looking as I do now, false eyelashes and all (which I figure would have made it all a rather ticklish affair). The fact is, I was born in the usual way on July 14, 1930, in Maryville, Tennessee, though my childhood was speeded up. I was six months old when I started traveling, I sang and danced by the age of 2, and when I was 11 I weighed 145 pounds, had reached my full height (5'5½"), had a 40" bustline, a 40" hipline, and a 24" or 25" waist. A terrific figure if you're 25; if you're 11, it can really get in the way. I was the only girl to flunk physical education three years in a row because I would not get undressed and take a shower with the rest of my classmates. They thought I was dirty, but I was the only person in class with breasts, and I was horribly embarrassed.

With boys it wasn't much better. There weren't any boys in my class, in the class ahead of me, in *all* the classes ahead of me, who were as tall as I was. They were all just about level with my bust. And when we had dances, with the girls always on one side of the gym and the boys on the other, the girls danced with girls and I always led. I had to lead, you know, I was taller than everybody. To this day, when I walk out on a dance floor, within three minutes the guy asks, "Who's going to lead, me or you?"

I grew up quickly. My father was a construction engineer, and since I was born in the Depression, we traveled on to another town every three or four months. I don't remember most of them, but they were Midwestern or Southern small towns, dreary and poor. I kept changing schools, averaging four or five a year. We were in Ohio, Indiana, Pennsylvania, Virginia, West Virginia, Florida, and Louisiana, to name just a few places. In one twelve-month period I attended ten different primary schools. If I found playmates, it was only to lose them, so it became much less painful not to make friends in the first place.

I turned to my mother for friendship. She was twenty when I

was born, a beautiful blue-eyed woman nearly six feet tall, with most of that height in her legs. She was always super-clean and smelled like face powder, though she wore little make-up then. She was as soft and gentle as her rich Southern accent, which she still maintains today. Once when she couldn't attend a school meeting, I was very upset. "Why is it so important that I go, Polly?" she asked me.

"Because you're prettier than any of the other mothers." She was. And she kissed me very tenderly.

My mother, Lucy, came from a family of twelve. Like my dad, she had little formal schooling. Her father had gotten the calling and become a Southern Baptist preacher, riding up into the mountains on horseback to preach. (He was never ordained, though.) He was tall, lean, very Lincolnesque, and measured 6'7". All his children were over 5'10". My uncle Bill was the tallest. He wasn't admitted into the Army because he had a size 15 shoe and they couldn't supply him. My grandmother was 4'10", with hair so long she could sit on it.

Mother, Dad, and I were a warm, self-contained family unit. Sometimes Mother stopped in the middle of housework to have a tea party with me. Or she would get down on the floor to play jacks. She ran the house and managed to be a little of everything to me. Dad's work kept him away from home for long stretches of time, and Mother was very strong (though less of a disciplinarian than Dad) and self-reliant.

Dad adored my mother. He was like a big, overgrown Irish teddy bear, 6'5", with dimples, prematurely gray, and totally godlike to me. I would have jumped off a twenty-story building for him. Fortunately he never asked me to do that, but he did ask me to be prettier than anybody else, get better grades than anybody else, be smarter, be better—and I tried to do it all for him.

If I had five A's and a B, my father asked: "Why did you get the B?" He believed "strong people don't cry," and when I fell down, he'd likely say, "Look, you left a crack in the cement." All my childhood illnesses were discovered in school, because I'd never admit that I was sick. Dad's insistence on strength might have come from the fact that his mother died when he was a child, and all the children were sent to an orphanage.

My parents were proud that I wanted to sing, but they never pushed. Dad did spend hours teaching me to sing along with him when he played the guitar. When friends came to the house (and my parents' friends were my friends, because I didn't have any others), inevitably the guitar would come out and my daddy would start to play and sing. By the time I was two I'd learned six numbers. If I was in bed and heard the guitar, I'd get up and join. But it wasn't that they urged me to. I never thought I had stage parents. Later, when I was in show business, I think my parents' main concern was that I wasn't sleeping enough and not taking good enough care of myself.

I was a precocious little lady, and very spoiled. Mother and Dad gave me almost anything I wanted. (If they didn't, I had temper tantrums.) Since my contact was with grown-ups, my vocabulary and behavior were adult. As a little girl, I was never really exposed to anyone my age. In that way, my life was like my idol's. And, like her, I wore ringlets (though my hair was much darker). Like her, I sang and danced for anyone and everyone who came to the house. At three or four, I knew that I was going to be Shirley Temple.

I was adamant; I wanted to wear only Shirley Temple dresses. They were extraordinarily feminine and frilly. I wouldn't wear any other kind of dress. I wanted to be like my idol. Dad never passed *his* dimples on to me, so I put clothespins on my cheeks to get them.

I wasn't aware that we didn't have as good a life as some other people. If my surroundings were sometimes grim, it didn't matter, because my world was a world of daydreams. I made up fantasies. Mother was incredibly kind, because she knew I was lonely, and whenever I talked fancifully, she backed me up.

I recall thinking my mother had told my father that somewhere along the way we were related to Dixie Crosby, who was then the wife of Bing Crosby. Dixie also came from Tennessee. Perhaps I dreamed that conversation.

But because I was desperate for other children to like me, and because I didn't know how to talk to them, since I was so seldom around them, one day I told everyone in school that Bing Crosby was my uncle.

The kids called me crazy and chased me home, throwing rocks at me and calling me names. That wasn't too unusual; they often did that, because I was one of the great liars among prepubescent human beings. But this time it wasn't enough that they chased me home; they knocked on the door and asked Mother, "Is Bing Crosby really Polly's uncle?"

"Yes," my mother told them, "it's true." Of course it wasn't. But Mom backed me up. (After the kids left, though, she warned me about doing that kind of thing again.)

My flights of fancy continued, spurred by loneliness. I believed there was something wrong with me, though I didn't know quite what. Later I didn't go on dates or attend football games or get invited to slumber parties.

My singing and dancing made the kids think of me as a showoff, and being an A student didn't help either. My teachers thought I was a ring-tailed wonder, and I could communicate with them much better than with my contemporaries. I simply didn't know how to make friends with people my own age.

It was easier to be a grown-up. At seven or eight I would secretly get out my mother's make-up and sit in front of a mirror, making sure no one saw me. There I transformed myself into a beautiful adult with lipstick, powder, and rouge.

I would dress up in my mother's clothes, and though every little girl does this, I think I began earlier and did it more often than most, even wearing her bras around my flat chest. I didn't really know who I was supposed to be. I never thought I was pretty, and I was more often complimented for performing than for my looks.

In fact, those compliments made me believe I was acceptable *only* when I performed. I knew I got attention when I sang and danced, and so, like a dog that gets fed when it does a trick, I came to believe that the trick, and only the trick, brought results.

For most of my life, that feeling stayed with me, making it almost impossible to zero in on who I really was. As an adult, I felt I was acceptable only as Polly Bergen, Singer, Actress, Performer, Entertainer, Show-Business Personality. Performing was my life, as a professional and—I realized quite late, through psycho-analysis—as a private person. My greatest personal problem has been the struggle to stop performing.

When I was nine, we spent a year in Circleville, Ohio. My mother was pregnant, and we stayed put until Barbra was born, even though Daddy couldn't live with us when he worked and came home only for weekends. I remember that town because I'd always wanted a sister.

Barbra was a beautiful child, but the difference in our ages was too great. My memories of her as a baby are that I couldn't go to the movies because I had to stay home and take care of her. I was a lousy sister, and had no patience at all. We've become close only in the last ten years. Now Barbra is tall (6'1") and, except for her eyes, looks exactly like my father. I, except for my legs, look exactly like my mother. Barbra married at the age of 15, when she had reached her full height. She later divorced, then remarried, and is now settled in Florida with two beautiful children.

I think Barbra had a tough deal being my sister. She always suffered from comparisons with me. At twelve, I looked eighteen. I had after-school jobs, was independent (Mother was busy with Barbra and Dad was on the road), and was singing professionally at fourteen. When I was fifteen and Barbra five, I was engaged to be married. So Barbra and I never had rivalry, but we also had nothing in common. And my successes, in school and as a performer, couldn't have made life easy for her. That, and her exceptional height, made Barbra become a clown. She had a delicious sense of humor, and being a clown was the easiest way of dealing with things. She still has her humor, but it's not so much of a defensive mechanism anymore.

A year or so after Circleville, we moved to Coraopolis, Pennsylvania. I was in sixth grade, the war was on, and my father was working outside Pittsburgh. We lived there only a few months, but I remember it because it was the first time I'd ever lived in a mansion. At least, it seemed a mansion to me. We were caretakers of the house and lived in our own quarters, but we used the living room, the radio, the piano. There was also a goat and a horse outside.

In Coraopolis I fell in love for the first time. He lived across the street in another mansion and had brilliant red hair and freckles. We played Post Office—the first time I ever played it. I lost. He kissed another girl and that was the end of my love affair.

It was there I read Shakespeare for the first time. The living room was like a library, and I read the little volumes of *Hamlet, Julius Caesar, The Tempest.* I loved them almost as much as my favorite radio show, *I Love a Mystery,* with Jack Webb, the best thriller on radio.

And another excitement: I got my period. I was riding the horse and when later I saw blood, I thought I'd hurt myself. I didn't tell anybody, and after a few days the bleeding stopped. My mother found the bloody rags and explained something, but we never had a frank discussion about sex, and I didn't know the facts of life until I was a senior in high school.

We weren't a very religious family, but my parents had been reared as Baptists, so I was one too. We went to church from time to time. I sang in church choirs and taught Sunday School when I was older, but I was never taught that the devil snatches little girls who put rouge on their faces. I was, however, totally ignorant about sex. And nudity, if not directly sinful, was certainly unattractive.

But I looked old enough to know it all. My physical development made me seem grown-up when I was still a child. I got jobs on the basis of gall (I always claimed experience where I had none) and looking old enough. I was a theater usher, drugstore clerk, model, waitress, car hop, and linotype operator.

My body and my sophistication gave me an advantage. I became aware that I could use my power as a woman. That power was a little frightening, but I used it whenever I could, to get a ride home from work or from school, to get free books from the bookstore if I sat on the storeowner's lap. I knew it was wrong and maybe a little dirty, but a free book was a free book and that was more important. It was a major discovery for a twelve-year-old, and a new aspect of performing.

I didn't notice other girls and didn't talk to them. Now, of course, women are a major part of my life, but I didn't have friendships with them until I was quite grown up. As a young girl, I copied movie stars: Lana Turner, Rita Hayworth, Alice Faye, Betty Grable—but my heroine was Ava Gardner. I wanted to be like her. I read movie magazines, copied the make-up and poses of the stars. I was going to be a movie star, I knew, and I wanted to look older, more glamorous, more sophisticated. My mother was no longer my model; now the sleek Hollywood beauties took over.

Mother and Dad trusted me implicitly and let me go my own way. I began smoking at fourteen to look older, and I still haven't stopped, although I've tried to kick this habit many times. (Smoking ages you quicker than almost anything else.)

At one job interview, the man looked up and saw a busty girl with dark hair poured into a black crepe dress that outlined her figure. The hair came below the shoulders, the face was hidden behind heavy pancake, the mouth was blood red. The blue eyes were circled with very black eyeliner, the lashes thick with mascara. A cigarette burned with blue haze. Innocent me at fourteen! The man probably thought I was twenty-four.

At thirteen, I was dating college boys. At fourteen, I was singing professionally in Richmond, Indiana, a place we lived in when Daddy was between jobs. We had many relatives there, and moved in with an aunt and uncle. I became engaged to marry a twenty-eight-year-old radio announcer. Shortly after the engagement (but not because of it), my family moved to Gardena, California, a suburb of Los Angeles.

My fiancé followed me there and found a job. On my fifteenth birthday he took me out on my first dress-up date, and I got very sick on sparkling Burgundy. Being nearly twice my age, he wasn't thrown by my behavior, and took good care of me. He was a warm, wonderfully considerate man. He was a sort of Jimmy Stewart type, tall, slender, and very handsome.

I was the only girl in tenth grade at Gardena High who was engaged to a grown man. We necked a lot, but I remained a "nice" girl. The engagement ultimately ended because of the age difference. I wasn't crushed, though. I was turning myself into a professional singer.

My first important job was as vocalist in the Dresden Room, a cocktail lounge in Hollywood. It was a respectable nightclub. Mother came with me, of course, and Dad used to chauffeur us there, sleeping in the car till two in the morning, when he drove us home. I sang at the bar, accompanied by a piano. The proprietors thought I was twenty-one and that my mother was my older sister. Actually, I was fifteen. The point is that I worked because I wanted to, not because we needed money. Whatever I earned I spent on myself or to advance my career.

During high school vacations, and sometimes through skipping school (it was all right, I kept up my A average), I sang in Las Vegas lounges with full bands. Mother came with me, but the musicians treated me like one of the troupers, patting my derrière, cupping my breasts, trying to get me to bed.

They didn't, but it wasn't for lack of trying. I was a torch singer now, and looked it. My face make-up was almost white, my hair was naturally dark, and I made up my eyes and lips to be very dark. The customers kept buying me drinks, but I wasn't of age so

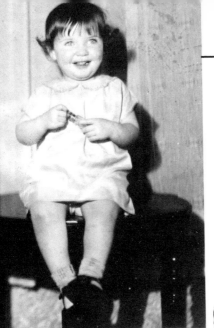

Here's how I got going

So all right, my childhood was crazy in many ways, but you can see that I wasn't unhappy or neglected. In the top picture I'm fat, cuddly, and one year old. The bottom photo is one that I really prize because my handsome father was rarely around and usually in a big hurry.

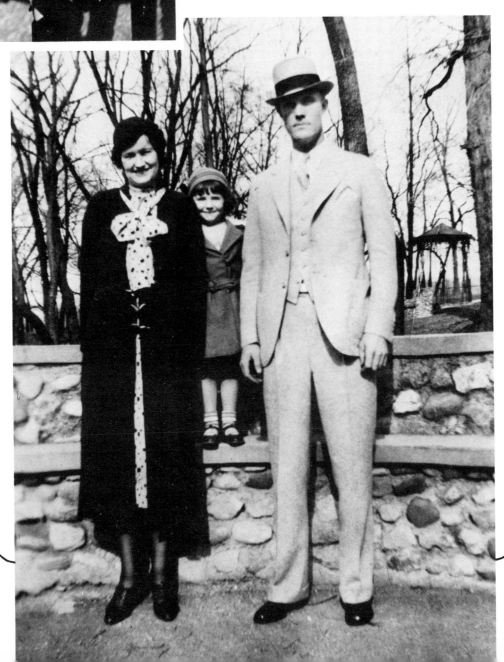

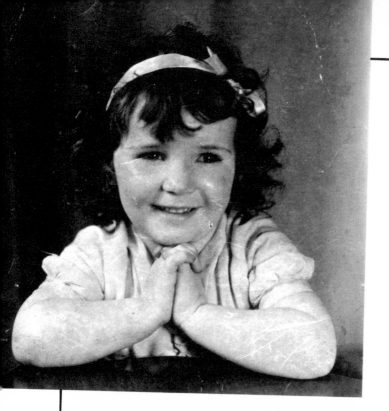
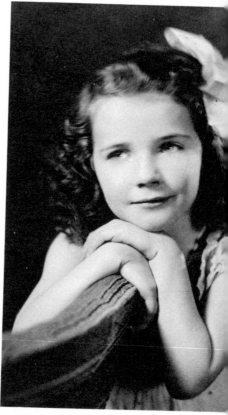
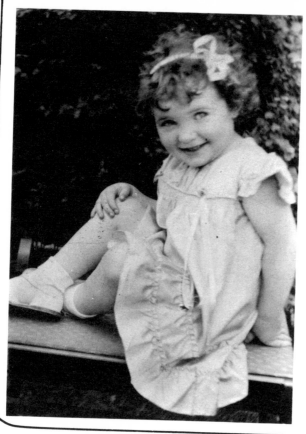
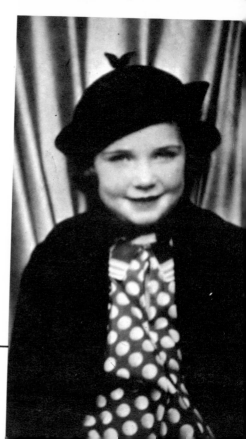

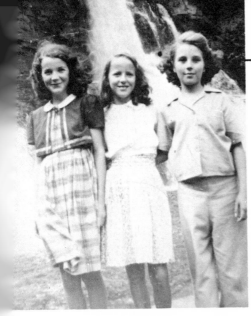

I started being a ham early. And as you can see from the four pictures on the left-hand page, taken between ages 2 and 7, Shirley Temple was my idol. Now look at the difference between me at age 9 (left, with boarding house neighbors who weren't really friends) and at age 13 (below), bosom and all!

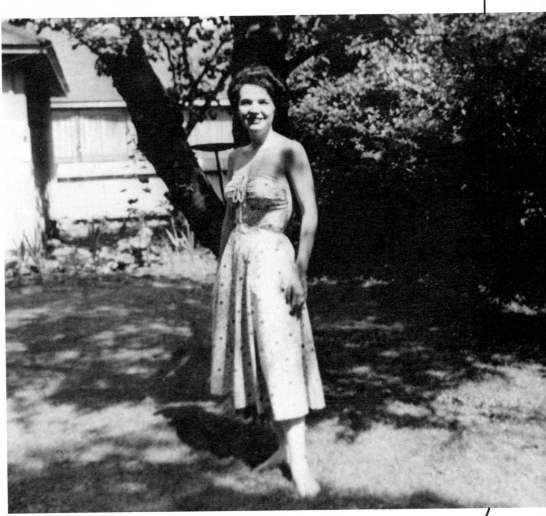

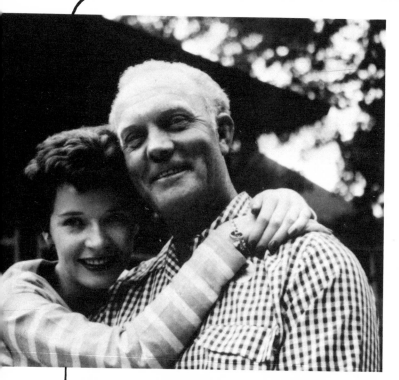

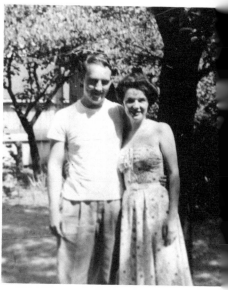

Daddy was like a god to me (top left) and came to my high school graduation (bottom). Mom (below) was more like a sister. I was shy with my first date (top) and incredibly naive and clean-cut in my first, busty movie studio publicity photos at 17 (right).

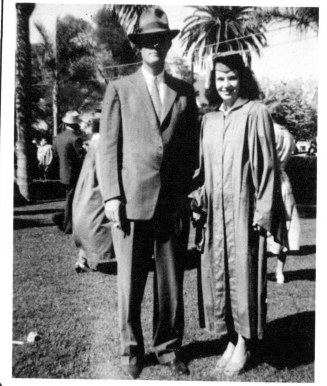

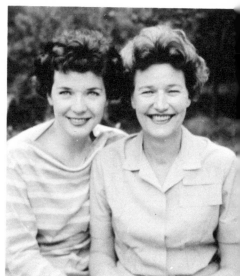

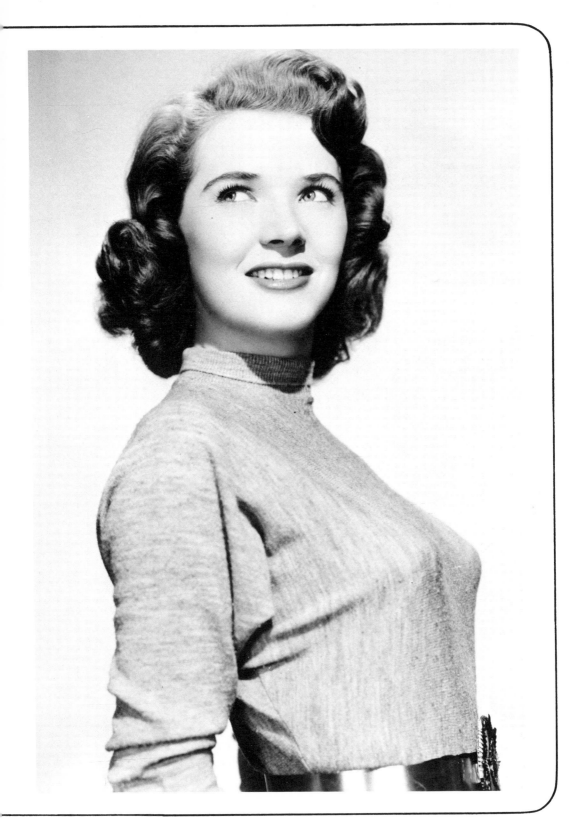

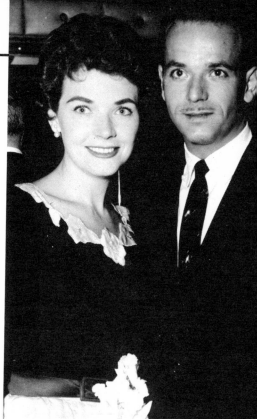

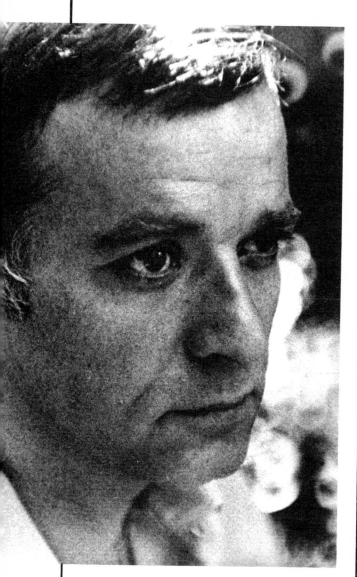

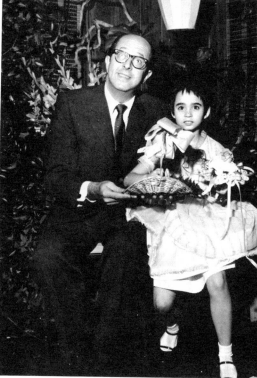

Meet my second husband, Freddie Fields, as he looked at our wedding reception (top right) and today (above). That's my daughter, Kathy, 9 years old, as flower girl at our wedding, with best man Phil Silvers.

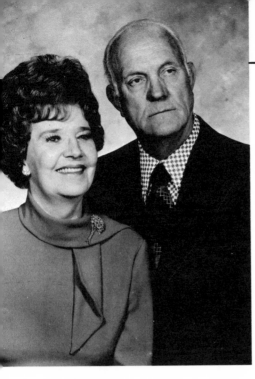

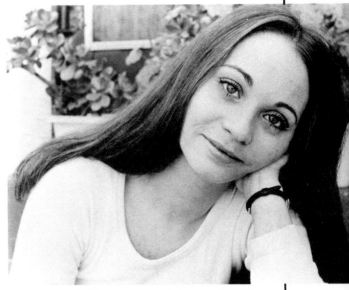
And here are my children today: (clockwise) Kathy, 26; P.K., 16; Peter, 14.

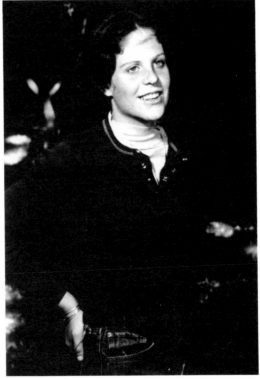

all-American couple: my parents in their
st picture, taken in 1973.

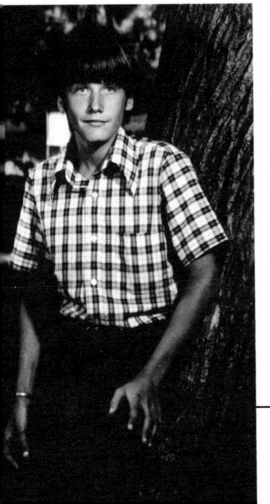

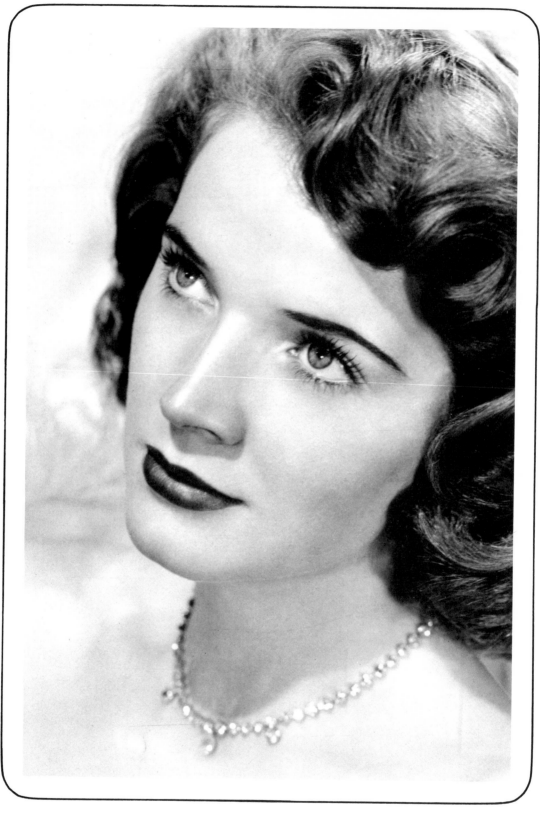

Innocent at 16 in a business that recognizes no innocence.

I handed them to my mother. She had to drink those in addition to the ones customers bought for her, thinking she was my sister. At the end of my singing routine every night no amount of white make-up could conceal my blush as I helped my poor mother out of the club.

My mother was getting bombed every night, but I couldn't let people know I was under-age. We had to think of something. We began pouring the drinks away behind our backs, into the plants near the microphone. It wasn't long before all the greenery turned brown and died, and the owners couldn't understand what was killing their plants. We never told.

A talent scout saw me perform in Las Vegas and recommended me to Sam Goldwyn as a possibility for his famed Goldwyn Girls chorus. Goldwyn always included scores of beautiful young singers and dancers in his film musicals. Lucille Ball and Virginia Mayo got their starts this way.

In the eleventh grade I quit school, assuring my parents I would return to complete high school, and went to Goldwyn Studios for a screen test. I was sure I would become a star. Yet, no matter what anyone says, nothing can prepare even a sophisticated girl for the process of becoming a movie star. Nothing. My experience in night clubs was minimal compared with the immensity of that prospect. Singing in a club and acting in movies is the difference between a bicycle and a Rolls-Royce. Singing in clubs is a way of earning a living; starring in movies is a way of life. In show business there is a strict caste system, and the Brahmins are motion-picture stars.

For three months I took singing and dancing lessons at the studio in preparation for the movie. I drove to and from the studio in my father's ancient 1933 Buick with the world's worst brakes. You had to start pumping them two blocks before you stopped. I spent a fortune paying off drivers I ran into.

After three months the whole production company fell apart —and I went back to school.

I finished up my senior year in six months, with my sights still on motion pictures. Singing in small clubs wasn't the way to hit the big time. Radio was the mass medium, and the best chance to gain recognition from the mysterious moguls behind studio walls. So radio it was.

I auditioned for several shows and then sang on *The Cliffy Stone*

Show, a popular radio program in Pasadena featuring country music and comedy routines. There was a young singer-comedian on that show called Tennessee Ernie Ford. I sang hillbilly songs, familiar to me because I was raised on country music. But I didn't have the simple, homespun voice that usually accompanies the lyrics and twangy sound. My voice was low and husky. I got fired by Cliffy after singing a lovely lullaby, "Go to Sleep, Little Buckaroo." Cliffy explained that, though personally he loved my voice, it sounded "as if you're trying to lay the kid, instead of putting him to sleep." He felt I should move into the pop field.

But I wanted to exploit the combination of offbeat voice and country music. My voice was sexy, with a grown-up, she's-been-through-the-mill sound. I cut some demo records for a small, now defunct label, KEM. One record was to make all the difference.

It was a number called "Honky-Tonkin'," a raucous hillbilly novelty song. I gave it a naughty, low-down sound. My manager sent a copy to every motion-picture producer and director in town, along with a picture of me in a sexy, low-cut gown with my hair swept to one side and long earrings. The combination of glamor and earthy sound did the trick. Hal Wallis, one of the most important producers at Paramount Pictures, liked the record and asked to see me.

I was terrified. I made up to look as much like the photograph as possible. At eighteen I still had baby fat. Hal Wallis had seen hundreds like me: pretty young girls in severe black dresses with make-up caked on their faces, their hair worn dramatically to make them look older.

He must have seen through all the fuss and feathers. He asked me to sit down and talk about myself, tell him my background as a singer and what I wanted to do in the future. He thanked me for coming in, and that was the end of it. As I walked out through the famous Paramount gates, I had a great desire to go back inside again. I was terribly discouraged, quite sure I'd made a bad impression.

Next day my agent called to say Mr. Wallis wanted me to make a screen test.

I remember I wasn't happy about the way I looked in the test. But Hal signed me to a personal seven-year contract with yearly options (his), paying six hundred dollars a week. It was a lot of money (it still is) for someone who hadn't acted in even a bit part. I was proud not to be a starlet—they earned one hundred fifty a week. I was already learning Hollywood's caste system, where salary was almost as important as the kind of roles you had and the sort of pictures you played in.

I made my movie debut in *At War with the Army*, with Martin and Lewis. The picture was a tremendous success, and I was stunningly forgettable. I like to think the reason for that was my appearance, my lack of experience, and a very small role—in that order.

To buttress my confidence and learn more about my craft, I worked with a singing coach. One of his students was a handsome young man making a name for himself as a contract actor at Columbia Pictures. He was the first man I'd ever met who was taller than my father.

He was 6′7″, his name was Jerome Courtland, and he was only four years older than I. He was fresh out of uniform from World War II, he had a beautiful body, and he was debonair. I was dazzled by him, though he was the youngest man I'd ever known. Our courtship was brief, and we were married in Las Vegas six months after I'd graduated from high school. My wedding dress was a white strapless organdy—which goes to show how much I knew about taste.

Jerry was dear, sweet, gentle, and adolescent. He was physically brilliant in everything, with the exuberance and gracefulness of a greyhound. He gave me the childhood I never had. We did dumb silly things together: making human-body pyramids on the beach, going to football games, doing all the things I should've done at fourteen or fifteen. When I married Jerry, he was like my first sleep-over date.

When we married, we were both earning the same amount. But Jerry came from a wealthy family. He'd never had to hustle, and I'd been hustling all my life, starting with baby-sitting jobs at ten. For Jerry, things had been very easy. At a cocktail party of his mother's, when he was seventeen, Jerry was discovered by a director and signed to a Columbia contract.

With Jerry, my social life changed drastically. The first time we went to his parents' house in Bel Air for dinner, I almost had a heart attack. I didn't know which forks to use—I'd never seen more than a single fork at a place setting. The house was beautiful and filled with rich furniture—I'd never seen anything but Sears-Roebuck furniture. I was a fish out of water.

Jerry's old friends were rough on me, except for Roddy Mc-Dowall, who was unfailingly sweet and kept saving my life. His other friends made me so uptight that I deliberately upset them. I would burst out with a four-letter word in the middle of a conversation because I couldn't stand all the put-downs I was being subjected to. Jerry was amused by my behavior.

But I learned. By watching Jerry's friends, Jane Powell, Amanda Blake, Elizabeth Taylor, Terry Moore, I realized I was wearing too much make-up and overdressing pitifully. I put away the black crepe dresses and got a sportier look. Jerry and I went shopping together, and he helped me pick out clothes. The Ceil Chapman outfits I'd been wearing had made me look like his mother, even though I was eighteen. Now that I think of it, 90 percent of what I learned about dressing, manners, and style was during my marriage to Jerry.

I made two more pictures, *That's My Boy* and *The Stooge,* with Martin and Lewis. They were superstars, number one at the box office. The movies were made inexpensively and the director didn't get in the way. Whatever the boys wanted to do was fine with him. His sole directions to me were "Roll 'em," to get the cameras going, and "Cut."

I needed a lot more help than that. I lost all confidence in what I was doing. And, to be honest, I wasn't very good. It was impossible to turn to Dean or Jerry. They were both relatively new to the movie business too, and in any case they were having such a good time clowning around the set every day that they hardly knew I was alive.

At that time I thought Jerry Lewis was the meanest human being I'd ever met. He was a noisy, self-centered man who constantly chased me around sofas—which he did to every pretty girl who turned up on the set. I think he did it just to amuse the rest of and cast and crew. Neither he nor Dean ever had any trouble with girls, who flocked around them because they were major stars.

Every day I was upset by the wild goings-on. Though as a band singer I was accustomed to swear words and a certain amount of vulgarity, my experience hadn't equipped me to deal with what

Jerry yelled across the set, especially when visitors were watching us shoot.

"Hey Polly, you old hooker, get your fat ass over here and see if you can read your lines" was about the nicest thing he said. Most of the time I worked with him I was on the verge of tears, or actually crying.

One night at a party of his, he said something—I can't for the life of me remember what—that made me burst out crying. I wouldn't cry in public, so I ran into the bathroom and sat on the edge of the tub, sobbing.

Tony Curtis came in. He was a big star at the time at Universal. I hadn't met him, but he put his arm around me and asked what Lewis had said. Then he comforted me, saying I shouldn't pay attention, it was Jerry's way and he didn't mean it. I always loved Tony after that.

Now I realize how unbearably insecure Jerry Lewis must have been, but I can never forgive him for being so inconsiderate.

Dean, on the other hand, was always easy to get along with and agreeable on the set. He was a gentleman, and impersonal, but I became awfully fond of him. When the team broke up, most people predicted that Jerry would go on to greater stardom and Dean would be unemployed. I loved Dean and disliked Jerry so much, I told everyone that Dean would be the bigger star. Happily, I was right.

Though I wasn't particulary happy being in Martin and Lewis movies, I got a raise and the future looked promising. Unfortunately, my husband Jerry's career was going in the reverse direction. Columbia was cutting back on production and dropped Jerry. He had reached his zenith before we were married. Now I was on the rise. Neither of us could have predicted it.

Eventually I broke my Paramount contract. I parted from both the studio and Hal Wallis on amicable terms. I wanted to star in big musicals and Paramount wasn't making any. Metro-Goldwyn-Mayer was, so I was advised to go to New York (such is the perverse logic of Hollywood) if I wanted to be discovered by MGM.

Whereupon Jerry and I went to New York, and I opened at the Maisonette Room in the St. Regis Hotel. The reviews were marvelous, and my hair, then a blondish-red poodle cut, earned me the title of "the apricot-thatched Polly Bergen." Jerry and I had a marvelous apartment on Beekman Place, but we weren't as happy as we'd been in California. I had started taking over, being aggressive; Jerry was retreating. That was to get worse, but we still loved each other and were young and hopeful.

After less than a year, I had an offer to play at Ciro's on Sunset Strip, the best club in Hollywood, and it was frequented by the MGM producers I wanted to impress. We left New York, which pleased Jerry, and returned to Hollywood. He was following my lead. But though I was still determined to be a movie star, I didn't want it at the cost of my marriage. If Jerry had asserted himself, we might have had a chance. But he didn't.

I was well received at Ciro's, and soon had my Metro contract. This was 1952, and the television scare had hit the major studios. The day I signed, mass firings began. Pictures already in production were reduced, and several movies on the drawing board were scrapped. Many musicals were thrown out the window.

As new girl on the lot, with only three pictures behind me, I was assigned to the studio's B unit. Metro made dozens of small, inexpensive movies to play on double bills with the blockbuster A features. In about a year I had worked in five movies. They were all acting roles, and I didn't know how to act—that should have been obvious to everyone. But I had no time to study acting: I was too busy being in the movies. I wasn't learning by doing, either, because the pace was too frantic.

My insecurities grew so overwhelming that I couldn't even watch the rushes, which might have given me some useful performance pointers. I didn't have the courage to see the movies once they were released, either. *Cry of the Hunted*, with Vittorio Gassman and Barry Sullivan, was the first. Then came *Fast Company*, with Howard Keel—the kind of movie that isn't expected to go anywhere, and didn't. *Arena*, with Gig Young; *Half a Hero*, with Red Skelton—and I was back where I started, playing the foil for a box-office comedian. I was going to leave, but was persuaded to take the leading-lady role opposite William Holden in *Escape from Fort Bravo*. At the last minute they decided not to take a chance on a newcomer and gave the part to Eleanor Parker. I had only a few scenes.

That was it. I was wasting my time, I wasn't learning how to act, and it was obvious to me I should be singing instead. I packed my bags, Jerry packed his, and we went back to New York, where I worked as singer on television shows. Movies had not been for me; I had failed, through my own insecurity. To succeed, you must want and push for stardom above all else. But for me, acting in movies had been a horrendous, emotionally debilitating, super-narcissistic job. I wasn't a good actress; I would never become a star.

In New York, Jerry was in a couple of Broadway shows, but they weren't very successful. I had my TV appearances and two Broadway shows. I was earning good money; I had a good agent, named Freddie Fields. Jerry spent a lot of time running down to Florida for scuba diving.

By now I had really taken over the masculine role in my marriage. Along with earning the money, I took care of the bills and made *all* decisions. I went out to look for jobs for myself *and* for Jerry. I decided where we went and what we did. When Jerry said something at a party, I jumped in and corrected him. If he told a joke, I tried to stop him. I ran the house, I ran Jerry, I ran everything. Jerry, in turn, was relying more and more on me. I began to lose respect for him and for myself.

I even told Jerry explicitly: "Whatever you want to do, I'll go along with you and be your wife and stop working. If you want to be a shoe salesman, fine. But I can do that only if you'll take over your role as husband."

Twenty years later, in a world of raised consciousness, that probably sounds silly. But it was my last-ditch effort to save the marriage. I asked for a separation, hoping it would force Jerry to get a job. It didn't. And in my male role I had lost the search for my own identity. I didn't want to be so strong, but the pattern was fixed. Jerry and I never fought. We'd loved each other in our own ways when we married, but as we grew up we seemed to go in different directions.

We divorced, and, curiously, our relationship seemed on better ground afterward. But within a few months Jerry told me, "I'm going to get married! I wanted you to be the first to know."

I smiled and mumbled something approvingly. Then I cried for six weeks solid.

A year later I married Freddie Fields. Freddie had been my agent as well as Jerry's, but Freddie and I paid no personal attention to each other. In fact, our relationship was sometimes strained.

Freddie considered me a television singer, not an actress, and every time I asked him about a chance at a straight acting part, he said simply: "Get out." Sometimes I really hated him. One night Freddie and I happened to be at the same professional function, and found ourselves talking for an hour, then two, then three, five—and three months later we were married.

He was an agent with Music Corporation of America (MCA), the largest and most influential agency for performers in the world. He was and is one of the brightest men I've ever known. He was the opposite of Jerry: Freddie was and is a forceful man, extremely strong. Too strong. He could (and can) handle any situation. He looked like a young Douglas Fairbanks, Jr. With Freddie I could forget about playing strong, acting the male. Freddie would take over and be my mentor. We married. His nine-year-old daughter, Kathy, was our flower girl.

From then on, Freddie was my teacher and critic, the man whose judgment I trusted most of all (except, of course, when it came to my acting). In fact, Freddie is the only person in my life whom I've completely trusted, been completely honest with.

It wasn't that he overpowered me—he was no tyrant. But he influenced me in everything: my clothes, my speech, my style of performance, selection of songs. I accepted his judgment and taste in most things. He was enormously creative and innovative mentally, using his humor to mask feelings and make devastating observations. He was responsible for my successes and for me becoming more desirable, prettier, sexy.

Being his woman and Kathy's mother made me regain my femininity. Kathy, who is now a miniature woman, was then a miniature child. Her face is all eyes, enormous hazel eyes. Her hair is very dark brown with touches of red in it. She was and is fragile, easy to break, a gamine. We always thought of her as a tiny bird; if we made too much noise, she'd fly away. I had a completely open relationship with her, and loved her.

Freddie and I tried unsuccessfully to have children of our own. I had three tubular pregnancies, each leading to a painful operation and heartbreak. Doctors told us it would be dangerous for me to continue trying to conceive. In 1957 we adopted P.K. (Pamela Kerry; Freddie wanted Pamela, which I hated, and I wanted Kerry, which he hated, so P.K. it was), and two years later we adopted Peter. Both were infants.

In 1957 and 1958 I had my own half-hour live television show in New York. This was offered to me after I had won the Emmy from the Academy of Television Arts and Sciences for "Best Actress" in the title and starring role in *The Helen Morgan Story.* That award had led to a dozen offers from Hollywood, but I turned them down because I didn't want to be on location, apart from Freddie and the children. I'd made a decision during the year I was divorced: Never again would I marry unless I met someone more important to me than my career. Not that I wanted to abandon my career, but I wanted a man with a stronger will than my own, around whom I could build a life.

Freddie was that. I could be big boss all day at *The Polly Bergen Show,* or do my stuff on *To Tell The Truth;* at night Freddie was definitely in charge. Much later I realized Freddie also needed my approval and support, as much as I needed his, but he was much less open about his needs.

We were both (as is everyone) products of our upbringing. We made certain assumptions, we went along with the world in many ways, and we were both anxious to be successful. Often, we didn't find the time or ways to be open with each other. And we weren't with the children enough when they were young. Freddie, especially, feels that now. Our youngest (Peter) is now fourteen, and when Freddie sees small children, he plays with them and reads to them in a way he missed with his own.

In 1961 I had been a regular panelist on *To Tell The Truth* for five years. Freddie decided to move west. It was a courageous move at the time—leaving the security of a large, going corporation for the risks of beginning anew in Hollywood. He formed Creative Management Associates, which was to become the most important agency of its kind in Hollywood.

We moved to a beautiful hilltop house in Beverly Hills, and almost immediately I was offered a top role with Gregory Peck in *Cape Fear.* I asked Freddie's opinion; he said to go ahead, it sounded like fun. After that one, I made *Kisses for My President,* with Fred MacMurray (I played the first woman president); *The Caretakers,* with Robert Stack, and *Move Over Darling,* with Doris Day and James Garner. I turned down twenty others because I didn't want to leave home and work someplace far off on location.

Those were happy years. For the first time I was fairly secure about my appearance, having finally established my individual look. My husband was terribly successful, our children were beautiful, I was considered one of the most important women on television, and Freddie and I were socially in demand. Our house was complete with theater, enormous swimming pool, breath-taking gardens, and beautiful furniture—a showcase house often photographed for a variety of publications.

In the house I entertained friends and stars. At one party Princess Grace came specially from Monaco; others jetted in from Europe and Asia. Frank Sinatra was there, as were Cary Grant, Rock Hudson, Lucille Ball, Rosalind Russell (in white lace), Raquel Welch (in halter top and mini skirt), and Ted Kennedy, then a very junior Senator, who was so unobtrusive that he was ignored.

I was having the time of my life. My Shirley Temple fantasies had come true.

In 1962 I made *The Caretakers,* a movie that changed me in many ways, bringing things that were deeply hidden up to the surface. I played the part of an insane woman, and because throughout my life I had controlled and concealed my emotions—I had *performed*—this role hit at something in me I was unable to handle.

Until then I hadn't realized my own coldness. I had no deep friendships, and I was frigid sexually. But I was an actress, after all, and able successfully to hide my frigidity from men. I also hid it from myself. After *The Caretakers* I went through years of therapy, during which time Freddie gave me enormous moral support. The first, intensive year made me open up to him more than I ever had, but it was already too late. We still had some good years left together, but I had been acting for so long, and Freddie and I had never confronted each other about the problems of our marriage. By the time I knew that something radical had to be done about us, Freddie's love for me had dimmed.

Our marriage was over. I had to go through the hard work of finding out who I was, as plain Polly Bergen, not as Mrs. Freddie Fields and not as Polly Bergen/Performer. The children were at a point in their lives where divorce was not as much of a trauma as we feared. P.K. and Peter were in school, both children whom we had raised to be self-sufficient. When Freddie and I broke up, we remained the best of friends. Whenever the children needed one of us or both of us, we were there.

P.K. is now sixteen and lives with me. She was a musical-comedy baby and is a larger-than-life teenager. Her hair is wild and russet, like a horse's mane, thick, shiny, and glorious. She has green eyes, and a peaches-and-cream complexion with freckles. She responds to everything at a three-thousand-decibel point, and there's no doubt that she's Sarah Bernhardt reincarnated. Cries from that girl have made us believe she was dying—she cries larger than life, laughs larger than life, hates and loves larger than life. She is your best friend or worst enemy; the coldest and most calculating, the biggest-hearted child I've ever known. She's totally sensitive to a situation or mood, and is the mother of the world. I spent her whole life saying, "P.K. you don't understand, *I'm* the mother, not you." No matter what happens to P.K., she'll come out on top. Both Freddie and I are very sure of that.

Peter, of all three children, is the most "inside." He is totally independent and very definite about what he likes, what he doesn't. His white-blond hair has darkened as he's gotten older, and he's a handsome, tall, lean boy. He collects rocks and stamps; he can take things apart completely and put them back together, often leaving out several things and still making it work. Like his father, he's not openly emotional, but he's a boy of great sensitivity—the kind of boy who, when he's grown up, will be capable of flying into outer space alone. And enjoying it, doing it perfectly, performing all his duties and never being lonely. Or, if he is, never showing it.

And Kathy is now twenty-seven, a gentle, soft-spoken idealist, a true romantic, and like many girls her age in love with her father. She has always needed to find someone who needs her, someone she can do something for. She is still the little bird that she was; she is still growing up.

I had to grow up after the divorce, and I couldn't use the children for it. I had advised Kathy not to become a recluse, and I wasn't going to be one either. I was forty-two years old, busy with The Polly Bergen Company (which I'd begun after *The Caretakers* and my retirement from the performing life), and the world was open to me.

I shouldn't have worried about my social life as a single woman. Available men cropped up from nowhere. I started playing backgammon seriously, entering tournaments and joining a backgammon club. The game fascinates and diverts me; it also brings me into contact with men, with people, I am interested in.

I've learned to be more free. I can go without make-up now, and my body pleases me. I'm more sensual than I ever was, and my former sexual problems seem to belong to another woman. Besides, getting to know and like myself, I'm going through a metamorphosis and becoming my own woman, belonging to no one but myself. I'm through with performing. I've learned to tell the truth about myself. My best advice to *you* is that you learn this for yourself, too. And in these pages, I'm here to help.

2

Imitation Is the Sincerest Form of Insecurity

You've decided to create an image, but remember: It should be of you. You will change, naturally, but then so should your make-up and hair. Your individuality must always be part of your look. It's the only thing you have that no one else in the world has, and no one else can compete with.

It took me many years to establish my own look. Early pictures of me at Paramount when I was eighteen never show the same girl twice. Here she's a healthy, simple, corn-fed kid; in the next, a sultry lady of uncertain years; then a bouncy sweater girl; an elegant, experienced woman; a debutante; an innocent from Queens or Brooklyn whose mother doesn't know she's out; or the mother of that girl. It wasn't until I was a regular panelist on *To Tell The Truth* that I locked into the "Polly Bergen look." It wasn't changed (though it was modified) even in movies I made after that.

As a girl, I took my mother as my model for looks. We were facially very similar, and in my teens people would think we were sisters, though our bodies were different, with her extremely long legs and my stumpy ones. You will find me supercritical of my legs throughout this book. This is still one area of self-criticism I have not *yet* been able to conquer. My mother wore almost no make-up and wasn't chic or fashionable. But she was beautiful, and I admired her a great deal. I've found that the relationship between mother and daughter is basic to a woman's attitude on beauty. If daughters admire their mothers a lot, they tend to copy them. And

21

the reverse: Girls who find their mothers unattractive often go to great lengths to look as different from them as possible.

In other words, the girl whose mother caked on too much make-up is likely to wear few or no cosmetics. The plain, un-made-up mother might have a daughter who goes the glamor route.

My mother was proud of my looks when I was a child. I never combed my hair, and once in a while my mother would take a few tranquilizers, pull me over to her, and spend hours going through the knots and tangles. But I didn't register my mother's pride. I didn't think I was homely, but I just didn't think of myself in terms of facial beauty. I thought of myself in terms of size and ac-complishment. Success was the important ingredient.

When I entered my teens, I wanted to look more sophisti-cated. I copied the stars in movie magazines, wore a lot of make-up, and did look older. My motive was to find jobs, and I suc-ceeded. When I was fourteen, I looked twenty, and Mother looked to be in her late twenties. Wearing very little make-up made her look younger; wearing a lot certainly aged me.

When I got my movie contract I also got a lot of other people's features. Every studio had its own stable of stars. The wardrobe, make-up, and hairdressing departments commonly used stars as models for youngsters. I wound up with Janet Leigh's eyebrows, Joan Crawford's mouth, and Marilyn Monroe's hair. (With my luck, it had to be *her* hair!)

No one designed a wardrobe for Polly Bergen, the unknown. So I was wearing hand-me-downs from Dorothy Lamour and Eleanor Parker, whatever was available. No one sized up my face and body for assets and drawbacks. My good features weren't highlighted, my bad ones not disguised. The specialists had preconceived notions and put bits and pieces, all unrelated, of other women on my face.

Naturally I was upset. I was miserable. But I didn't make any objections, because I had no idea what to do about myself either. I didn't like my appearance, yet I was too unsure of what I wanted to make a fuss.

Hal Wallis thought I had potential, but he left the details to the experts. Each department worked on me independently of the others. I was attractive—not truly beautiful, but not ugly. Non-descript, somewhat chubby. My baby fat gave me a Mae West type of figure: large breasts and hips, small waist. The Marilyn Monroe syndrome was in full flower then, and every young actress was given a version of that look. I see now that I was something of a Grace Kelly type, cool-looking and best without much make-up. But my timing was off, a little too early. The put-together, ladylike look hadn't quite arrived.

The first time I asserted myself about my appearance was during the filming of *The Stooge*. It was a period piece, and the head of Paramount's hairdressing department was determined to put an old-fashioned hairdo on me.

"We'll give you a nice marcel wave, honey," she told me. "Like they did in those days."

"That's what you think!" I snapped. "I've looked bad enough in those dumb hairdos you gave me in the other two pictures."

"You don't understand about movies, Polly. Everything has to fit the time period and the costumes."

I bit my lip, trying to control my temper. I told her there were times when you had to forget authenticity, especially when it interfered with the actor's appearance. "It looks God-awful," I said.

"You'll wear it the way I fix it," she insisted. And I did. She was a diehard.

The hairdo was absolutely terrible, and I was upset for days. It was a short bob, with a part on the right and a marcelled wave. Horrid. I look at still photographs from that picture and don't recognize myself.

I soon left Paramount, and in New York I learned about fashion. New York women were much more chic than Californians in dress and make-up. At twenty I was able to absorb everything, but I had no personal identity, no distinctive look of my own.

Later, on my return to Hollywood, Metro gave me dark hair. I was still a conglomeration of many stars, and there was no definitive Polly Bergen image. In the eight movies I did, I couldn't have been recognized as the same girl twice. The only thing that was characteristic of me was that I didn't wear false eyelashes. All the other actresses did. But I had a reverse ego going; I tried desperately to believe I was pretty, and that meant I had to look good without such obvious artifice.

Television make-up in the late fifties was very heavy and cakey to compensate for the extra bright lights. On *The Polly Bergen*

Show I wore a lot of shading to hide my plump face. I was fifteen pounds heavier than I am now, so I learned to keep my clothes simple and uncluttered—no bows, no jewelry near my face.

David Lawrence, my make-up man, showed me how to achieve a natural look with a minimum of base, eyeshadow, lipstick, and rouge. By the fourth or fifth show we had decided to include a torch moment: a closeup that framed my face from a point just above my eyebrows to a point just above my chin. No one had dared so close a closeup before. I couldn't move my head even a fraction of an inch without moving out of the light or disappearing from the lens. With the camera that close, it would have been insane to wear heavy make-up. The focus was on my eyes, and even though television was all black and white in those days, people got the message of vivid blue.

On guest appearances and dramatic shows, I experimented with my own look in make-up, clothes, and hair style. A dramatic show I did with Henry Fonda on the *General Electric Theatre* not only taught me a lot, it set in motion the underlying theme of this book.

It was a story about a woman with scars that disfigured and distorted her face—and changed her personality. The way she looked altered her completely. That show had a far-reaching effect on me. Afterward I visited women's prisons to talk to the inmates about beauty: how to dress, make up, and do their hair when they were released to society. They could improve their lives by changing their appearance—I believed it firmly then, and I believe it now. I feel that most women who get into trouble are terribly insecure, the sort who drives the getaway car simply to please a man.

An insecure woman doesn't believe she's beautiful. And a lack of beauty, or at least a woman's conviction that she is not beautiful or attractive, can ruin her psychologically, and that in turn can destroy her life. It's the point of this book: Looking good is feeling good. If you're pleased with your appearance, you're pleased with yourself and with the world.

On television my hair was finally done my way, and so was my make-up. Studio experts no longer dictated what I was to look like; I had a distinctive look. The only thing that bothered me was that I had to wear glasses. I'd had to most of my life, but I didn't want to. So I left off my glasses and developed a squint, a furrow over the bridge of my nose. On *To Tell The Truth*, I toyed with my glasses on camera, sneaking them on when the camera was directed at someone else. When the camera returned to me, I'd grab them off my nose and twirl them in my hand. It became something of a signature with me.

I had my own look, but I was afraid to relax it. I wouldn't have been caught dead by friends or strangers without being totally put together—all the make-up, perfect hairdo, and the rest. I was Polly Bergen, but I still didn't know what a Polly Bergen was. I thought it was my appearance that made me acceptable. I lived in the reflections of others, particularly Freddie's.

He made me feel desirable and attractive. But when his attitude began to change, I didn't know what I was. Though both my husbands had told me I was beautiful, I didn't know what that meant. No matter how often a man tells a woman she's beautiful, she won't be convinced until she can make that statement to herself.

I've learned now to relax a lot. I can go most anywhere without make-up and without my hair done. The old rigid woman is gone for good. When I'm doing business as head of The Polly Bergen Company, I'm almost without gender. I'm a female executive, without sexual connotations, and I can wear the old Irene Dunne hairdo to look neat and efficient.

But I can also put on a pair of studded jeans, a turtleneck sweater with no bra underneath, go barefoot, and feel eighteen years old. Or a slinky crepe gown and feel I'm the sexiest woman who ever walked into a room. It doesn't matter if others don't agree with me; that's how I *feel*. If I go to a formal, black-tie party I wear quite a bit of make-up. At a less formal one, I leave out foundation and lipstick. At an intimate get-together I'll wear almost no make-up at all. But I have a look, and whatever one it is, it's mine and nobody else's.

Every woman in the world can and should create her own look. So many of us exist with a kind of fear, an insecurity about ourselves, that we compete with other women. That is a fast way to destruction. In competing with another woman, we are trying to live up to her and outdo her. How do we outdo her? By doing whatever she's doing, only better. And we end up with imitation. Bad imitation.

When I sell my cosmetics, I emphasize that no woman should buy them because she wants to look like me. All she can hope to be is a second-rate Polly Bergen, and that's nothing compared to being herself: that special woman she and nobody else is.

Everyone has this ability. A friend who could most charitably be called horse-faced, is the hit of every party she goes to. She's a woman with a great brain and powerful job. She has a sense of style that's completely her own, not eccentric but elegant, electric. She'll come to a party in a high-necked, long-sleeved black outfit with an incredible belt and a fantastic piece of jewelry on her shoulder or at her waist. She has a great sense of humor, a wonderful intellect, and she's dynamite. She comes across as beautiful.

On the other hand, I remember one time Jerry and I were going to pick up Elizabeth Taylor for a party. We waited half an hour, then forty-five minutes. We were going to be very late, and I was impatient. So I went up to her room.

It was a mess. Hairpieces were scattered all around. Thousands of dollars' worth of clothes were spread over the room; the vanity was spilling over with make-up and treatment products. Elizabeth was looking into her mirror.

"I'm not going," she announced. "I'm ugly."

Poor Liz! I thought that on her worst day she's maybe as ugly as Grace Kelly. But we were getting later and later, and I told her she looked great, and could she just hurry up.

I thought I'd convinced her. But at the party something was off. She didn't feel right, and she was sending out vibrations to everyone at the party. The most gorgeous woman in the world wasn't beautiful that night. It's the woman *herself* who makes beauty happen.

This has a lot to do with establishing your own look. It doesn't mean, however, that you should necessarily stick to a way of dressing or making up all your life. I've seen celebrities hang on to the look that prevailed when they rose to fame. Marlo Thomas, for example, still wears the same huge eyelashes she favored in her television series, *That Girl.* The long triple sable lashes worked for her on the series, but they're so overwhelming, I can hardly see the rest of her. They're also hopelessly outdated.

Ann Miller's age is pinpointed by her make-up. She hasn't changed a thing since she was first fixed by a make-up artist at MGM in the early forties. She still has the very dark, vivid red mouth, the darkly accentuated eyebrows, the white skin, and the masses of hair that were very popular in 1943. Women date themselves with old make-up habits.

It's a matter of experimenting, being flexible about yourself. What works for one woman may not work for you. What worked ten or twenty years ago might not work now. Establishing your look means emphasizing what is special about you.

Total self-confidence is a goal that very few people completely achieve. But once you've done your best in make-up, hair, nails, and dress, and are happy when you look in the mirror, you know you're *there*. When you go out the door, you should leave all thoughts of your appearance behind you. It's like preparing an automobile for a trip: Once it's been serviced and checked, there's no point spending the whole trip worrying whether something will break down.

The woman who prepares herself, who's learned the best hairdo and make-up for herself, makes it clear to everyone that she is who she is, and likes what she is. Illusion can bring out the reality of you.

3

Stand Naked

Do just that—in front of a full-length mirror in a strong light. You can do this alone, or with someone. (Personally, I prefer to lock the door.)

Look at yourself critically. Certain things will almost surely be apparent to you. If you like what you see, fine. You're a lucky one. But if there are ten, twenty, seventy, a hundred pounds too much of you, you'll have to do something. You could get a new mirror. (Maybe the kind they have in circuses and fairs.) Or attack the problem directly.

Nakedness in broad daylight (if you're not in bed with a lover) can be tough. I know. For years I couldn't bring myself to look at my own naked body. My Southern Baptist upbringing was definitely Victorian about the human body, and nudity was not acceptable.

Four years ago, things changed. I looked at my reflection in Freddie's eyes and saw a blur. I thought I was getting old and unattractive—undesirable. In self-defense I bought all sorts of negligees and sexy nightgowns. But they didn't set the reflection right. I became terribly self-conscious about my body.

Then one day, fortified by a glass of white wine, I did a meticulous striptease in front of my bedroom mirror. Slowly I removed my clothes, piece by piece. Removing my shoes was the greatest wrench. I don't like my legs, and the high heels made them look longer and better-shaped than they are.

I studied my body critically, first as a single entity, then inch by inch.
Naked, I wasn't in bad shape, but I wasn't the most devastating
sight in the world either. I wasn't really looking for the attractive
points; I was looking for the facts. All women, I suppose, *sense* their
physical shortcomings, but out of an instinct for self-preservation
they keep those thoughts at the back of their minds, and don't try
to conduct the inescapable self-investigation.

Face to face, it's hard to fool yourself. I now study my body in
the mirror every day. So should every woman. The reflection may
be hard on the ego, especially if breasts sag, buttocks droop, and
there's a flabby cushion where the waist is supposed to be. It
doesn't help either if thighs look crepey and loose, the abdomen
wrinkled and stretched; if there's a matron's hump on the back,
varicose veins in the legs, and drooping flesh under the upper
arms.

Don't despair! *Make a list.* Write down your drawbacks and
get them out of the way. Then list your assets, *all* of them, including facial features, hair, breasts, shoulders, hands, waist, feet, legs.
When you look at the lists side by side, you realize what you want
people to see and what you'd rather they didn't notice.

The lists let you deal with the positive elements while simul-
taneously handling negative ones. "OK," you say, "I have a bad
neck but a wonderful mouth." Then it's a matter of learning to
dress and do your hair to cover the lines of your neck or to make it
look longer or shorter. A short neck looks longer if you wear a hair
style away from your face and neck, perhaps upswept. Lower
collars and necklines also lengthen the neck. (If your neck is too
long, you could reverse the procedure, but I never saw a long neck
that wasn't an asset.) Then you make up your mouth to be the
center of attention.

I'm oversimplifying, of course, but the jigsaw puzzle of one's
body is put together slowly and with great care: accepting this,
rejecting that, trial and error all the time. No matter who the
woman is, she has some feature working for her, and she can make
it really work. An incredible mane of hair. Exquisite eyes. Hands
that are absolutely beautiful.

I'm sure that when Barbra Streisand looked in the mirror in
the early days, she felt that she was a disaster area. But she had a
wonderful voice and incredible hands. And when she sang, her
hands moved all the time; you listened to the voice and you

watched those long, long fingers, those fantastic hands, and as the evening went on she seemed prettier and prettier. And as Barbra became more secure, she moved her hands less, and established a look that was completely hers. Now, because of her, many girls aren't getting their noses bobbed, and she's become a great beauty.

Every woman can find something to work on. Let your face go naked too. I don't wear make-up when I look in the mirror. No false advantages; start off with *all* the bare facts. Don't overlook your teeth—they really show. Unattractive teeth can ruin the entire look of a person's face, and I know people who never smile because their teeth are so bad. On the other hand, beautiful or distinctive teeth can be a focal point, even if the mouth is not particularly lovely. Gene Tierney's slightly buck teeth helped make her a great individual beauty.

With teeth, the sooner you do something about them, the better. It's vitally important for overall health in later years. All my children had bad teeth, and they all wore braces and night braces. I had to scream and yell at them every night to put them on. But today they all have beautiful teeth. All parents should take care of their children's teeth, and train them to take care of their teeth. If parents do nothing else (and I don't care if you're on welfare, then take your child to a clinic), they must correct their children's bad teeth.

If you're grown up and have terrible teeth, it'll cost you a lot of money. There are root canal and capping—all sorts of involved and expensive dentistry. But it's generally worth it for the final appearance. The whole mouth can be rebuilt, without pulling teeth. Generally speaking, false teeth should be considered only when your own become a health problem, when they *have* to be pulled because of abscess or whatever. If your teeth are yellow, or not as white as they should be, you can use teeth whiteners. Also, a very bright lipstick with a strong blue color makes teeth look whiter.

All right, I'm lucky, I have good teeth. But the first thing I saw in the mirror were my short legs. Next, my indefinite waist, which proved a blessing: By concealing my waist I could make it look higher than it actually is. That gives me the illusion of having longer legs. I complete the trick by adding high heels, and my legs appear four or five inches longer. Amazing!

The next thing was my torso. It's so long that when I sit, I seem to be over 6 feet tall. I've danced with men a foot taller than myself and then looked at them eye-to-eye at the dinner table. All my leading men, including Gregory Peck, who's about 6'3", had to have pillows placed under them when we were filmed sitting down. When people ask my height, I tell them: "I'm five foot five and a half inches. Five foot five of that is my body, and the half inch is legs."

But I have to accept that. No point slumping in my seat to convince my dinner partner I'm petite. Foolishness. And at times there's also a limit to how much I can disguise my stumpy legs. The high heels are great, but they look sort of strange when you're naked, and they feel rather peculiar in bed.

When a woman's faced with the impossible, she should accept it and make the best of it.

Now the mirror tells me my derrière is too low. (You want to know how I see it in a full-length mirror without breaking my neck? Easy: Standing with my back to the wall mirror, I look into my hand mirror, and study my back as carefully as I do my front.) My behind is underslung. Some women like that look—I hate it.

But I also despise girdles and corsets—too constricting. So there's no way for me to change the shape of my fanny through artifice. I have to rely on clothes again. Form-fitting skirts are out. In this Time of Trousers, I can buy pants that don't hug my hindquarters or cling to my buttocks but still look chic.

I have to shop with great care and use ingenuity. There's usually a label in the pants that says "Front." I turn that around and get in backward. The front, which is supposed to be flat for the stomach, works perfectly in the back for my flat behind. The back part, which is roomier, fits perfectly in front over the part where I'm supposed to be flat but am not. It's marvelous how things can work for you if you're willing to try something a little different.

I don't have a problem with my shoulders. They're extra broad, but that doesn't bother me. I like broad shoulders. Mine aren't bony, so I can show them off in evening gowns. Having broad shoulders lets me carry more weight than most women my height. My face is broad and my head big for my general appearance. The broad shoulders balance them off.

Some parts of my body, as with other women, are not good but not bad. They're just all right. My upper arms, for instance, are not flabby, but they're not beautiful. My breasts have always gone from very good to fair. They don't sag or droop—and in that respect I'm lucky. They depend on how seriously I work at exercising, but I admit I'm proud that, at forty-three, I have breasts with uplift and firmness.

Studying my abdomen and stomach confirms my suspicion that neither is as flat as I'd like. On the beach at Acapulco, the girls never have a tummy. They're built the way I'd like to be. That's typical, I guess: wanting to look other than you do. But it's a real waste of time. Dreams of looking the way someone else does should fade in the bare light of reality. I tell myself that.

In my lectures to women around the country I've wanted to tell them: "Look. Be happy with what and who you are," but I know they aren't going to be happy, because they haven't reached a point where they can like themselves. Not yet, at least. But it's a point everyone *can* reach.

Once a woman realizes there is no point in measuring herself against some preconceived ideal, it becomes easier to accept herself. There is no absolute so far as the female form goes. (Though if there were, I'd say Raquel Welch would be pretty close to it. But she probably has found a part of herself *somewhere* that she wants to improve.) And everyone can improve some part of herself.

I don't worry about parts of my body that I can change through diet and exercise. I just have to apply myself there. But body structure is something else again.

Some defects can be changed. I check for any trace of crepeyness just beneath the line of my buttocks. Every day I examine my legs for the first sign of troublesome veins. I overlook nothing. I inspect my stomach to make sure it hasn't developed a crease.

I'm equally meticulous about weighing myself daily. Changes in weight mean my body will probably look different. If I gain four pounds, I can bet it will show up where it'll be seen, on my body or face. Perhaps my stomach will pooch out a little—just enough to be noticeable in my new pants. Sometimes my stomach will pooch out a lot. There may be a little bloat to my face that wasn't there before.

There's nothing I can do about my ankles. They're too straight; they don't curve enough. I inherited them from my mother and I'm stuck with them. I can't change their shape. But I usually wear dark hose and higher heels than are in fashion, so my ankles appear to have more shape.

My trouble is that I'm essentially a perfectionist. I'd like every physical aspect to be (or at least *seem* to be) flawless. This means, of course, settling for less. It doesn't mean getting hung up on your good points, though.

If a woman's too fat, she mustn't kid-herself. Either she's pregnant and should go to a gynecologist—or go on a diet. It does no good to tell herself that her husband, lover, or children like her roly-poly. Probably the one who likes her obesity least is the woman herself.

Bad posture shouldn't be shrugged off either. Positive and quick action is absolutely necessary, and not just for appearance's sake. It can affect health; many back pains and foot ailments stem from bad posture. The very worst things I had going against me were my posture and my lack of gracefulness.

As a child I was a lump. When I reached my full height at eleven, my coordination resembled that of a Great Dane puppy. I did everything I could to conceal my height. I wanted my breasts to appear less huge (my bust was forty inches when no other girl in my class had even peanut-sized breasts), so I even tried binding them. Of course I developed horrible posture, and until a short time ago I thought of myself as cowlike and awkward. Or horse-like. Yes—I sat, walked, and leaned against walls like a horse. Pretty faces are so easily come by in Hollywood that they simply aren't enough to give a woman self-confidence. That's how it was with me. I had a pretty face, not spectacular, but it couldn't be isolated from the rest of me.

An attractive face will make a great first impression. The impact is terrific if you want to go to bed with a guy—once. But a more lasting impression, or relationship, takes more than a good face. A pretty face can quickly become as boring as a plain one if the girl doesn't have more to offer, as I've made clear enough in the preceding chapter.

When I take off all my make-up, brush my hair flat, and stump around, I'm not an ugly woman, but I'm not exactly startling. I see myself as an ordinary, plain, nice-looking female. But the moment I straighten up, hold myself well, and move gracefully, then I am something more. And so is every woman.

Exercise is largely responsible for my improved posture. Exercise and concentration. I've concentrated on holding in my stomach so well that it's become an unconscious habit. Now I can be perfectly relaxed and at ease and my stomach remains flat. (Well, almost flat.)

By sucking in my abdomen, I naturally thrust forward my chest, and my shoulders fall back naturally. As a result, I sit and stand erect. I appear to be proud of who and what I am. I can still breathe properly *and* hold in my stomach. Eventually the reminder to hold in my stomach has a psychological effect. If I look proud, I feel proud. And that's not the same as vanity.

Some woman will follow my advice, will take off her clothes, and stand smack-dab in front of the mirror. She will see a five-foot five-inch woman with sagging breasts, fat behind, short-waisted trunk, pitted skin, terrible nose, bad teeth, skinny legs, and forty years of wear and tear. What then?

Then she begins one thing at a time. It's never too early to start beauty habits, and it's certainly never too late. Why should a woman accept herself if she doesn't like what she sees or the way she feels? Preposterous! If she wants to improve herself, she will. When an active person stops working, she finds herself falling to pieces. The same is true for the woman who gives up on her appearance. Retirement from oneself will bring the same loss of lust for living that retirement from work brings.

This woman must say to herself, "Somewhere in this absolute mess is a lovely person. She can look lovely too." And something will work, as soon as she's working for herself.

Be cautious of experts, though. They're selling their products. The hairdresser has his services to sell. It's easy for him to tell a woman she'll have a fantastic head of hair—if she puts it in his hands. The manicurist is out to sell her on how beautiful her nails can look—if she comes in twice a week.

Some specialists can be pretty objective. I think I am. I know I can be unbearably honest with women. If a woman is fat, I say: "You're fat."

I'm not hurting her; I'm doing her a big favor. That's the best thing anyone can tell her. And I don't pull any punches in telling her the truth. "You may be able to fool yourself, and even a lot of other people," I tell her. "But I'm telling you you're fat, and that there's no reason in the world today to be fat." I let that sink in a moment before I clinch it: "There's no such thing as being too thin. No woman can be too thin or too wealthy."

Of course, you *can* be too thin, but it's a good line to throw at a woman who's fifty or a hundred pounds overweight. I've found the phrase sticks with women and bolsters their determination to lose weight.

The man in a fat woman's life is usually her biggest problem. If an overweight woman is married or has a lover, that fact alone can give her sufficient security to remain obese. He tells her, "I love you the way you are." So she does nothing. She thinks, *Hey, he loves me as I am. So why should I lose weight? Maybe he wouldn't love me anymore if there was less of me.*

Maybe, just maybe, the man in her life is fat and feels less guilty about it if she is too. Maybe, just maybe, that man in her life feels he looks better because his woman is hefty. By going along with it, she is pandering to his cruel ego.

But fat people will find any excuse not to lose weight. They will go to any lengths to avoid dieting. Any rationalization is brought in to avoid the torture—and it really is torture—of losing weight.

The fat problem can be overcome. Almost all the physical difficulties I've mentioned so far can be overcome. Or repaired, or disguised. The main problem is that few women, even attractive ones, have the vaguest idea of how to deal with themselves. So many women come off as plain and settle for that.

The seeds of beauty lie in almost all women. But they must be willing to recognize and work for it. Hundreds of thousands of women, millions of women, are too lazy.

American women are more free than any others. The way to use and enjoy that freedom most is to be beautiful and confident. The reason for being attractive (another way of saying "beautiful") is to please. Ourselves first, then other people. Getting beautiful for a man is nonsense, no matter who the man is.

We should be beautiful so that we feel better about ourselves, and more free. Women owe it to themselves to be beautiful for themselves alone.

4

...And You Can Do It Anywhere

It isn't necessary to find a gym or a swimming pool or a golf course to practice this fun sport. You don't have to travel in search of snow or sun. You don't have to dress for it. You don't even have to have a partner (though personally, I prefer one). Sex can be done almost anywhere. It's certainly as good for you as tennis, and it takes a lot less equipment.

A few years ago I would probably have stopped this chapter right here! But times have changed, and I hope I've changed with them. (I also hope my father has changed, or doesn't read on.) Because sex and beauty can't—and shouldn't—be separated. For sex is a beauty consideration—second only to love. Sex is an attitude, a frame of mind, the physical appearance of sensuality. It should be developed and blended with the rest of a woman's characteristics to make her the most vital sort of woman she can be.

For too long, false modesty and rigid upbringing have kept us from this aspect of true beauty. For hundreds of years women have been encouraged to conceal their sexuality. The female body was elevated to art in sculpture and paintings, but in the flesh there was taboo or shame connected with it. Even now, though the female body is being exploited in movies and magazines, it often is tabooed on a private, one-to-one basis. I think it's time we faced the part sex plays in our attractiveness, and go on from there without a blush, giggle, or cry of dissent.

Inhibition itself is unwomanly and, I think, unbeautiful. I

36

know because I lived with it most of my life. There was shame in the body, in its shape and size, its hair, smell, and texture. But a woman isn't just a brain or a face or a heart, she's one whole being. And no definition of beauty is valid that doesn't take in the body. There's beauty in a female athlete on the court or riding a horse. There's beauty in the way a woman walks, in the tilt of her head, in the body's attitude.

No matter how brilliantly she talks or how perfect her features, it's her body—limbs, torso, breasts, buttocks, shoulders, abdomen—that fills out the total picture of beauty. Unless and until a woman is comfortable with her own body, she can't claim to be beautiful, and, therefore, neither can anyone else think her beautiful. If she doesn't respect her own body, neither will the man she loves.

She must force herself to be unselfconscious about all aspects of her body, yet positive about what she feels is good. The more attributes she's proud of, the more beautiful a woman becomes. Beauty does *not* lie in the eye of the beholder—it's only reflected there.

How else can the seemingly unmatched couple be explained? I've known dozens of married couples where one partner was incredibly attractive and the other a total failure in appearance (at least from my point of view). But their definition of beauty was in the total person.

Or maybe it was the sex factor. Every woman has heard one man say to another, "What does he see in an ugly woman like her?"

"She must be marvelous in bed," the other suggests, and they both accept the explanation.

A real extension of beauty is a woman's joy and willingness when she enters into sex play. Her attitude is a thousand times more valuable to herself than to her lover, though he will reflect it. But if she has freed herself from conditioned passivity, she can find security and happiness in the fact of being a woman. In other words, *she is fulfilled and beautiful.*

I feel that the role of sexual submission is outlandish. Why should any woman assume it simply to please her lover if, in the process, she displeases herself? It's an affront to womankind.

But I'm a fine one to talk. When a senior in high school, I was sitting on the back porch with a girlfriend and finally got up the courage to admit I didn't know how babies were made or what the sex act was. I didn't think I was typical of my generation, and for years I'd pretended to know everything because I was so embarrassed at knowing nothing. Partly my Baptist upbringing was to blame, and partly it was that I looked much older than my years and pretended I was forty. No one told me the facts of life, because they were sure I knew them. I was an outcast in things sexual.

As a woman, I wasn't so much ashamed of the sex act as intimidated by it. In both my marriages I was a borderline case of frigidity. I didn't welcome the thought of sex; I tolerated it to please my husband. A most unbeautiful state of affairs. I didn't like myself for it, but I wasn't able to speak up about it.

Sexual misunderstandings and frustrations are the major cause of divorce, and the number one reason for unmarried couples to break up.

Sometimes a woman is a pleasing sex partner only until marriage. Afterward she doesn't cuddle quite as often, respond quite as readily. If her husband runs his fingers through her hair, she's likely to be annoyed that he's messing it up. He thinks of love, she thinks of the hairdresser.

I say to that woman: Let him muss up your hair! If it means you're late to a party, terrific! Don't go to the party at all. What's more important to you, your man or the party?

I forgot those things when I was married to Freddie. I felt that I had to arrive on time wherever I was supposed to go in order to please people who, for some unfathomable reason, seemed more important to me than my husband. I wasn't aware of it at the time—I didn't tell myself I was choosing a dumb party over Freddie—but if he got home late from the office and people were expecting us, I made him feel guilty because I worried that they would be angry.

Now I'd realize he must have had a rough day to be coming in so late. I'd figure, if we're late, we're late. If they're angry, they're angry. Too bad; other things are more important.

And it's the same thing if a woman withdraws when a man reaches to touch her or kiss her. She wants to preserve her makeup and "look right" for him, instead of responding to his instinctive gesture. What good does it do him to see beauty, react to it, and then be told he mustn't touch? I don't mean a woman should please someone else instead of herself. Not at all. But by pleasing the man you love instead of frustrating him, you are also pleasing yourself.

Woe to the woman who turns her lips away because she's afraid her husband will smear her lipstick! Imagine that he would turn away from your kiss because he had just shaved. This is rejection of a high order.

When I get off an airplane and know somebody demonstrative is going to meet me, I'll have just a touch of color on my mouth and some lip gloss, so I won't look pale and wan, but not so much of either that it will end up all over his face. I'm very conscious that I want him to kiss me. I know that now—I learned it too late for Freddie.

But I did always know better than to put a lot of cream on my face at night. Few things turn off a man as quickly. Instead, I apply a night treatment that isn't greasy and has a pleasant smell.

Creams, treatments, chin straps, curlers, and the similar horrors have no place in bed. In fact, I don't know anyone who wears curlers anymore. There's no excuse for wearing them. They scare the hell out of men. And women who wear curlers in stores or on the street are a disgrace to themselves. If you must use curlers, pick a time when you're alone—without even the mailman or the telephone repairman around. Or use hot rollers, with conditioner. I do, and it takes only a few minutes to have a really good set.

At night there should be no obvious beauty ministrations; they interfere with sensuality. I believe nudity is marvelous. If you like your body, it's provocative for both of you to show it off. Every woman should do it often. Admittedly, it's great fun to get into a really exciting nightgown once in a while, but I think women who wear old unattractive nightgowns or pajamas do it on purpose.

If a woman doesn't like her body but her husband does, he should let her know and help her to feel good about it. When she understands that, she also may get to like her body. I'm finally at a point where I'm free about my body—no more hangups. Years ago the male body was almost unattractive to me. Now I find there isn't any part of a man's body that I don't like. I love to touch him when I care for him. I get enjoyment from the taste of his body and the feel of it. It's a sensuous pleasure seeing my man undressed or undressing, and I enjoy having him see me naked too. I like him to take pleasure in the sight and feel of me.

Women have a tendency to grow lazy or forgetful about sex. "It's time to go to bed," they think, and prepare themselves to go to sleep. But once in bed, things might change. A woman's body should be pleasing, to herself and to the man. Even when I'm tired or sleepy, I like the feeling of my body being desired, being wanted.

That doesn't mean I douse myself with heavy perfume or make up my face. No. After my evening bath I rub on a soft body cream, knowing the sensual feeling I get out of it will be shared by the man in my life.

But I never wear a deodorant to bed. The men I know are turned off by deodorants. Personally, I don't find any natural body odor offensive. Heavy perspiration, yes, that I don't care for. But I like the light perspiration that's part of love-making. I love the feel of a wet body.

There's something sensual, intimate, and beautiful about exploring a man's body and having him explore mine. I like to feel the softness of his armpit, for instance, with its private and natural fragrance. That arouses me; strong underarm deodorant doesn't.

Sometimes I wear toilet water sprayed lightly on my arms, around my breasts—but not *on* them. (Even if the smell is delicious, the taste won't be.) I spray it on my legs and *around* the genital area. But I believe there's a natural feminine odor that's exciting, and I don't want to disturb it.

Any woman who's in doubt about what her man likes about her body, or what excites him, shouldn't be subtle about it. *She should ask*—there's nothing wrong with asking! If he likes her to have hair under her arms, she should let it grow unless it's repellent to her. I'd let it grow now if it were important to a man, but I wouldn't have said that when I was married to Freddie. A woman should consider these little things and use judgment of her priorities.

What does hair under the arms have to do with beauty? Well, stop and consider the pleasure it may give you and the man you love. Why should a shaved armpit be any more or less attractive than the natural look? On the other hand, if body hair is unattractive to you or him, why not shave the genital region? It's all a matter of custom.

While in this area, another problem can come up for the woman who douches too frequently. The natural vaginal odor is a strong aphrodisiac for both men and women. It should be. Men are generally excited by it, a fact that's difficult for many women to accept. But when the woman is aroused, this aroma becomes a sexual stimulant to her too.

Nobody should use crotch deodorants. Number one, they're a waste of time, since the distinctive female scent is internal anyway; and number two, they can be quite dangerous, causing burns, irritations, or infections in a very sensitive area.

Some women prefer to use dusting powder as a scent and drying agent against perspiration, especially in delicate areas. That's fine, as long as it's not directly on the genitals.

Men don't have to worry about that. Personally, I prefer a man without deodorant. I like the scent of the male and the scent of the female, that very personal identifying aroma. Smell can be more offensive than taste, texture, sound, or sight. A disagreeable odor can turn people off faster than anything else in a relationship. But smell is a part of beauty and of relationships. If we all wore the same deodorant, we'd be eliminating an important part of individuality.

But I do use an antiperspirant (which I apply every fourth day), because I perspire very heavily in certain areas. This compound, prepared for me by a pharmacist, has no commercial name. It is a 25 percent aluminum chloride solution, is odorless, and any pharmacist can make it up for you. But it *is* very strong.

I like having a distinctive scent, and I use only one fragrance. The chemists for my company experimented with 383 formulas before they came up with "Tortue." Perfume is a personal matter, I feel, and should be noticeable only when you're getting personal. It shouldn't set off an alarm or announce the wearer three blocks away.

A fragrance changes from woman to woman. It blends with the natural body oils and the woman's own aroma to create a different fragrance on each body. But the general aroma can be recognized without destroying individuality. "Tortue" is fresh, green, earthy, ferny, with a foresty fragrance; it isn't too floral, and carries with it a sexual note. I use the toilet water behind my ears, on my neck (front and back), my arms, around my breasts, my stomach, thighs, and back. I dab the perfume behind my ears and between my breasts.

When a woman uses fragrance to turn herself on, she turns

the man on too. It's just one of many little things. Something else a woman should do, I think, is to read a couple of pornographic novels. She can learn a great deal from them. Nasty? No, only if we've been preconditioned to believe that any graphic description of the sex act is a one-way ticket to hell. Juvenile? Perhaps, but even if a sex book doesn't excite the woman, it can be informative. For one thing, they're almost all written by men, so they give women an inkling of what really arouses a man. Writers of pornography take bodies and sex organs through flights of fancy into incredible turn-ons. Reading these books can reassure a woman and leave her more open to experimentation, because she knows other people are doing and thinking about what's in her fantasies.

Experimentation is the renewal of sexual fulfillment. It can be small things, like painting your nipples with lipstick. That's fun. Pornography is useful for dreaming up bedtime adventures to combat whatever monotony has crept into the relationship. But a woman should be honest enough to ask, "Did you like that?" If he didn't, OK, nothing lost. But if he did, then both partners have something new to look forward to in their sex life.

There should be more sexual dialogue between a man and a woman during love-making. Sex shouldn't be just executed, any more than a face just made up. Sex should be talked about between partners, but not treated too seriously either. There's a lot of sex talk, some of it indirect, among unmarried couples—that's the way it should be. But often it stops when they marry. Couples talk about vacations, parties, bills, meals, and everything else in the spectrum—why not the enormously important subject of sex?

If talk during sex is exciting, a woman should learn how to talk. She should use the vocabulary of explicit sex terminology. And she should learn to make her voice exciting. Not even a homely face turns people off as much as an unattractive voice. And I know women with such spectacular voices that they overcome ordinary faces and seem to be beautiful.

The first time I heard myself speak, I was astonished—and not pleasantly. It was in the days before tape recorders, and I heard it on an old-fashioned wax recording. I sounded like a man, a male Martha Raye. I had one level of pitch and volume. Though I'd made use of my voice for years in singing, in conversation I had almost a monotone.

Something had to be done. I went to my friend Phil Silvers,

and that wonderful comedian went to work on me. He is a perfectionist, in timing, in getting his punchlines through with emphasis, and in delicate nuances of inflection. He never reads a line the same way twice. He's always experimenting, and uses his voice as a musician would use a delicate instrument. I listened to him as if he were my voice instructor.

He taught me to use inflections (the rising and falling tonal qualities) and volume. I discovered the voice can be used and manipulated, and its proper use will make almost any subject more interesting. The more musical range there is in a woman's voice, the more people will want to listen to it.

Today I have a tape recorder. It's a good, cheap investment. I listen to myself to make sure I'm not slipping back to sloppy speech or the old monotone. I want to be able to use my voice like a musical instrument when I'm talking with people or giving speeches. Listen to your voice. Does it add to your beauty or take away from it? Put more color in your voice; make it a lovely thing.

And then talk about whatever you please. But don't forget sex. Talk while making love can be very arousing. Try it if you haven't done it before. Marriage should be the beginning of exciting sex, not a leveling-off period. Sex takes time to reach a special intimacy of body and spirit. That sex makes a woman beautiful.

I've heard more than one man say that sexual desire in a woman's eyes makes her more beautiful than she ever imagines. I think it's true. The flush of love or desire or passion is a tremendous look. Actresses try to bring this expression to the screen. There's an adventurous, abandoned *something* that catches fire in a woman's eyes and sets her skin aglow. Why should she try to hide it?

The first contact a person has with another is visual. There's no way in the world to believe looks don't matter. They do, for both sexes. And a woman should think about her closeup appearance when she's getting herself together. Closeup is what really counts when the introductions are made, so it's better to look your best at a distance of two feet than at ten or more, across the room.

Maybe I feel that way because I have bad eyesight and must move in close when I talk to people. I've been told this is very intimidating on my part. But a closeup look at a man is important to me—and to him.

My attitude is freer now than it was. The way I carry myself, my make-up and hair—I'm simply not "put together," as I was during my marriage to Freddie.

If a woman is too well put together, men are wary of touching her, afraid they'll mess something up. They think she'll react in an uptight manner. A woman should look touchable, messable or mussable.

When Freddie and I were married, I'd come home at night, take off my make-up and clothes, have a bath, and go to bed. It took me a long time to get ready for bed, to undo my look of the evening and prepare for tomorrow's look.

Now I go out and we end up at the man's house. We begin to neck. And what in tarnation am I going to do with my false eyelashes? Do I say, "Wait a minute while I take off my eyelashes"? And then, what about my make-up? Or my wig? What's he going to do during that time, read the paper? recite the multiplication tables? or just go to sleep? It's all a great argument for the undone look.

I'm also against wearing girdles, corsets, iron-maiden bras, and the rest of the armor. I prefer to wear no underclothes at all. That has nothing to do with exhibitionism. Freeing myself from binding bras and panties that ride up gives me comfort, first of all. It's wonderful to move easily within whatever garments I wear.

Secondly, it's sensual. There's something special in knowing your body is unencumbered by restrictive clothing. I feel proud of my body as it is; then the texture of my clothes takes on an almost erotic quality.

It's especially effective under crepe or jersey clothes. When I wear pants, I use shields for sanitary reasons. If I can, I buy pants with shields already sewn into the crotch. These can be taken out, washed, and easily sewn back again. In the summer I wear very tight pants, and the Visible Panty Line (VPL) is an unflattering thing to see. If the pants don't have shields, I buy them at a notions counter. If you can't find pants shields, use arm shields. Adjust them, sew them in, snip, and wash. It's not a big deal, and a lot better than wearing panties that show. In winter I wear body stockings that don't show seams or ridges.

There's nothing wrong, of course, with wearing figure-controlling garments if a woman needs them or feels more comfortable wearing them. Many women with large or heavy breasts are uncomfortable without a bra, and I wouldn't dream of persuading them to go braless. Underclothes today can be so feather-light that you almost feel you're wearing nothing.

It's important to shop carefully for undergarments and trust the salesperson. Certain kinds of bras and girdles can be damaging. Girdles with extremely strong control have a tendency to make a woman give up trying to control her body. If they're worn constantly, her muscle tone falls apart. I know that if I'm wearing uncomfortable clothes, if they're too tight or restricting, I become less agreeable. Who doesn't? A girdle that takes the smile off your face may be doing you a much greater disservice than a sagging stomach. Beauty is fine, but not at the cost of extreme discomfort or unhappiness. Anyhow, I can't think of many women who look beautiful while in pain. Uptight clothes make for an uptight woman.

When I was my put-together self, without a stray hair, with my face done up and my nose powdered, wearing an exquisitely well-made dress, my attitude went along with that compact, tight appearance. As I've freed up inside, so I've relaxed outside. I've discovered men prefer me in a loose jersey shift, wearing less make-up and with my hair loose. I become more touchable, more real, and, honestly, more sexy.

It's important to like your own body and show that you do. I'm proud that people can see I'm not wearing a bra.

This is a big change for me. For most of my life I couldn't make love with the lights on. Now I don't like to make love in the dark. I like to see what I'm doing. If the man turns the lights off, I'm secure enough to turn them back on. I tell him: "I want to see you." Sight is part of eroticism.

I like men who are bright and quick. I prefer tall men, but height isn't all that important. Sometimes I'm first attracted to a man because of his appearance, but some men are too good-looking and turn me off. And fat men don't attract me. (I don't mean to insult the beefy brigade, but I am conscious of male bodies now and fat is offensive for me.) I like a man with a suntan, with healthy color in his face. Not the white, white indoor look—I suppose that's why I'm not often attracted to Englishmen.

I see nothing wrong with men trying to look their best. I don't mind if they wear toupees or use bronzers or hair color. If men use moisturizers or skin balms, fine. They shave every day of their lives, and need something to soothe their skins. Also to soothe mine.

I could fall in love with a man who didn't make a great deal of money. I just rarely meet one.

I still haven't outgrown the please-the-man syndrome, but that's because it pleases me. It's fun.

Sex should be fun, free and inventive, *not* a ritualistic exercise. It has to be approached with a sense of humor. Ultra-serious sex can be very heavy and displeasing, defeating its own purpose.

Sex should be enjoyment of oneself, and through that enjoyment of another. Without sex, a woman develops tight lines around the mouth and her nerves are shot. Looking and feeling sexy doesn't have to focus on sexual gratification itself; it's an enhancement of beauty, a way of being. Sensuality transforms all parts of the body—toes, armpits, fingers, the whole body. A toe is just a toe, but when it's singled out for attention it becomes beautiful. I know.

This may be the first beauty book that says it, but sex and beauty go together. You can't be beautiful outside if you're not beautiful inside, and I'm not just talking about the mind.

5

Shape Up

Show me a woman content with her figure and I'll show you a seven-year-old girl. Everybody else is engaged in the war against flab.

In this push-button century we live in, excess caloric intake is no longer worked off by scrubbing, bending, stooping, and reaching. We don't have to do the back-breaking work that once kept us reasonably slim. Yet we no longer look fifty when we are still in our twenties. June may be in our faces, but our bodies are busting out all over.

Exercise is vital to good health and beauty. In my opinion, it's more important than all the make-up and hair preparations put together. The secret of its success is circulation, bringing blood —and therefore oxygen—to all the cells of the body. But exercise is a boring subject to many people. If you're one of those, skip this chapter. If you're not going to do the exercises, there's no point reading about them.

Many women apply an exercise program to their housework, stretching to dust high places, bending in the proper way, dancing behind their vacuum cleaner, or whatever. But nothing, I find, is as effective as organized calisthenics. Not even sports, though they're fun and beneficial. I play tennis, ski, swim, and ice skate, but I do none of these on a regular basis, and regularity in exercise is all-important.

My best period for exercise was when I had *The Polly Bergen*

Show on television. Each show included a dance sequence, which required an hour or two of rehearsal every day. Never in my life have I been in better shape.

These days I haven't the time to devote an hour or two to dancing, or any other exercise for that matter. Most women in this country don't have the time either. But it is possible to take out fifteen or twenty minutes a day for exercises that will do the job.

Set a definite time every day for exercise, and stick to it come hell or high water or burst pipes. I do my exercises in the morning. If I'm busy I adapt my schedule and do them in the evening. While traveling on business, I make sure to run through my calisthenics even if I'm in a hotel room. Let's face it: a room's a room!

When I don't exercise, I'm tired in the morning, no matter how much sleep I get. I don't enjoy my food as much as usual.

Curiously, when I'm tired and in need of a pickup, I find that fifteen or twenty minutes of exercise do more for recharging my batteries than anything else. I can feel the tingle of circulation in the tips of my fingers and toes, and the prickle just underneath my scalp.

Exercise can help specific body problems. Once, when I had forty-inch hips, I was able to take the weight off my hips through spot reducing. Also, I can add two inches to my bustline. It can't be done in a day, but I have the exercise that does the trick. I'm able to reduce the measurements of my buttocks and upper arms. I manage this by following exercises given me by Marvin Hart, a masseur and exercise authority. I started working with him years ago and have never had serious worries since. Marvin worked with Errol Flynn to keep him swashbuckling for those movies he made. Marvin's the reason Jack Benny looks so firm and youthful. Raquel Welch is a product of Marvin's almost magical exercises. Marvin himself is in his sixties, but looks in his forties, thanks to following his own advice.

Before I give his exercises, a word of caution: *Any woman unaccustomed to exercise should consult her family doctor.* Under no circumstances should fat women exercise without seeing their doctors. Fat turns to muscle with heavy exercise and is then twice as hard to get rid of as it was before. Maybe your doctor will advise you to begin slowly and easily, perhaps just walking a mile a day until you've built up your strength.

The most practical thing to wear for calisthenics is a two-piece cotton sweatsuit—the plain old gray, drab kind is warmest and best. It helps you work up perspiration and is easy to launder. But you can work out in any loose-fitting garments that don't restrict movement or circulation. Pants are fine, but not skirts. Panties or shorts and bra are all right in hot climates; otherwise, it's better to wear clothes that cover arms and legs, to retain body heat and discourage chills or muscle cramps, which come from fast evaporation of perspiration.

A slantboard costs about twenty-five dollars, sometimes less, and is the best exercise investment of all. The frugal woman can pad a bench top and get almost the same results.

Never use a bed for exercising. The mattress and springs have too much give and can cause serious harm to your back.

When you're ready to start on the exercises, begin with this warm-up. It has five steps:

Step 1. Lie prone (on your stomach) on a flat padded surface. Roll the body first to one side, then the other. While lying on your left side, raise your right arm and right leg, so that fingertips touch toes at a right angle to your body. Then roll over while lowering your arm and leg; repeat the exercise on your right side.

Step 2. Lie on your back, bend your legs in toward your tummy, and clasp your hands together underneath your knees. Flex legs from the knee, up and down. This tightens the back of the thighs and strengthens the knee joint.

Step 3. In a standing position with legs far apart, place one arm straight up in the air alongside your head, the other arm straight down alongside your thigh. Now bend your waist from side to side. Reverse your arms and repeat. This exercise is especially good for the inside of the thighs.

Step 4. On the floor, prop yourself up on your elbows and knees, face forward. Lift and extend one leg up behind you, raise it as high as possible, then lower it almost to the floor, and finally return to your original position with both knees on the floor. Extend and raise the other leg.

Step 5. Sit-ups can be done in two ways. Either: (1) Sit and stretch your arms full length out over your head. Touch your toes, with

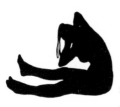

arms and legs extended. Or: (2) Sit. Clasp your hands behind your head and bend to touch knees with your elbows.

Both versions can be done on the bare floor, on a carpet or on the backyard lawn. They're most effective when done on a slantboard, which holds the feet down. Sit-ups strengthen stomach and abdominal muscles, as well as the thighs, calves, and back.

The total warm-up shouldn't take more than five minutes. Go carefully at the beginning, to avoid pulled muscles and soreness. Gradually increase each exercise until you're comfortable doing a dozen or more of each.

For the general exercises, always begin slowly at first and build up to the point where you are comfortably doing two or three sets of each repetition—that can be thirty of each exercise in all.

Now for the abdomen: Using a slantboard or bench, lie on your back and bring the knees up to the stomach while holding firmly to the back of the board with both hands. Stretch your legs straight out as far as they will go (don't let them touch the board) and point your toes. Hold that position for a count of five, then bring knees back to the stomach on a count of five, and stretch them out again, without having them touch the board.

This exercise strengthens the body from the waist down, tightening muscles and firming up flab.

For the neck: Still on your back, slide up on the slantboard, or lie flat on a bench, and allow your head to hang over, suspended. Keep chin horizontal, without lifting or lowering it. Keep mouth open and relaxed. Now tip your chin up slightly, toward the ceiling, allowing head to drop backward. This exercise is a great improvement over the old-fashioned version of raising the chin as high as possible and then lowering it, which stretched the skin. Keeping it rigid on an even keel strengthens chin and jaw while adding firmness to the skin.

Here's a real body toner for abdomen and stomach: Sit high on the slantboard and anchor your feet under the strap. Fold your hands over your chest, then lean backward slowly as far as you can go.

Straighten up to sitting position. I do this exercise in three sets of ten—that is, thirty times in all, resting after each ten.

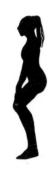

A tough exercise for the stomach is often the best. My favorite or at least the most effective, is to stand up straight, legs slightly apart. Put your hands on your thighs, and keeping trunk straight bend knees slightly. Bring your stomach in and lift it. Hold for a count of ten. Beginners won't get to ten at first; they'll be lucky if they can breathe. But after a while you'll be able to hold your stomach in for a count of twenty. Then relax, walk around a bit, and return to the exercise again. It's really isometric and has fantastic results. You're pushing your stomach against gravity.

The bust builder: I'm told again and again that it's impossible to increase the bust by exercising. That's simply not true. It can be done; I've done it, and every woman can do it.

Many years ago I had a severe illness and lost twelve pounds in seven days. My breasts disappeared on me. They lost inches and drooped. But by exercising I firmed them and added two and a half inches in the cup (*not* the back).

Of course, it's true that the actual breast doesn't increase. Neither the mammary gland nor the fatty tissue gets bigger. What the exercise does is build up the pectoral muscle *underneath* the breast, pushing the breast up and out. We see this in male weightlifters and body cultists. A favorite pose of the male physical-culture buff shows his chest bulging with pectoral muscles, giving him unnaturally large "breasts."

Those same muscles can be built up and maintained by women who want to increase their bustline. It's just about foolproof. And this exercise not only enlarges the bust, it's a wonderful way of reducing the upper arms while relaxing tightness in the shoulders and lower neck.

The bust builder is guaranteed if done religiously.

Lie flat on your back with your head at the top of a slantboard. Take two five-pound dumbbells (three pounds if that's all you can handle), one in each hand. With palms facing each other and elbows crooked, lower the weights to your sides. Now bring them back toward each other with little jerking movements until your arms form an oval above your chest.

Imagine you're making a basketball hoop of your arms; that's how you slowly bring hands in together right above your breasts. Return hands to your sides. The dumbbells add necessary weight and strain to work on those underlying pectoral muscles. No movement should be too fast. Repeat this exercise twenty or more times once you're used to it.

This particular pectoral exercise also builds up biceps, those muscles along the top of your upper arms which men like to show off by "making a muscle" for their awed children or flattering girlfriends. Biceps are often flabby and unattractive on women. So try the dumbbell exercise—and watch the sag disappear.

In the beginning, try each exercise only two or three times. *Nothing* will discourage you from exercise like sore muscles.

All exercises, in fact, should be started gradually. It's an old maxim among athletes and calisthenic authorities that the slower you go, the faster the results. Too much jerking of the muscles breaks them down instead of building them up.

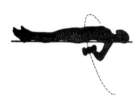

Another upper-arm exercise: Lie on your back with your head at the top of the slantboard. With your arms hanging down, hold dumbbells at your sides. Lift them from the wrist and elbow, with palms turned toward each other. The hands, in a clapping position, never meet, but come to rest over the chest. You are exercising your triceps, those long muscles at the back of the upper arm. As we age, this area tends to lose elasticity and the skin hangs. This is the ugliest problem women have with their arms.

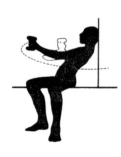

Another good breast exercise: Sit on the slantboard with your legs on either side of the board. Have a friend, husband, masseur, or whoever sit behind you. Lean against him (or her). (I do this with Marvin.) Hold weights straight out in front of you with palms inward and a slight curve in the elbows. Draw the dumbbells in toward you, holding the chest out. Bring weights forward again without lowering elbows, your hands coming together to form a flat oval. Move arms out to the sides as far as you can without losing the bend in your elbows, then back in again. Your arms should remain on the same horizontal plane throughout.

This exercise is great for building the major pectorals, but it works *only* if you use dumbbells (or something else weighty), three- or five-pound ones.

Once the exercise has been mastered I suggest three sets of fifteen or twenty per workout. Everyone has a different potential for building up muscles. Some women have to work longer and harder than others. I may be one of the lucky ones who don't have to work so hard. If circumstances force me to skip exercising for a time, I need only five or six workouts to snap back in shape.

For hip reduction: In a standing position with legs firmly apart, place your right arm straight up in the air and your left straight down at your side. Raise left arm, bend it around the back of your head, and grasp the elbow of your right arm. Now bend as far as you can to the left, moving from the waist. (This puts pressure on those pads of fat on the hip.) When you are bent as far over as possible, hold for a few seconds. Straighten up slowly. Repeat ten times, then reverse arms and do it ten times on the right side.

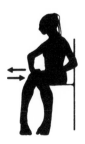

For the lower pouch on the outside of the hip: Lie on your side on the floor on a towel or slightly rough blanket and swing legs backward and forward in a stiff-legged scissors motion. Hold for a few seconds. Be sure the center of the pouch of fat is getting the full weight of the body. The lower the lump is located, the lower you should hold your feet to ensure pressure is on the right spot. Be sure to wear clothing in this exercise, preferably lightweight trousers, to prevent skin burn. Repeat scissors exercise thirty times for each leg on each side.

For excess fat and flab on the inside of the thigh: Sit erect at the edge of an armless chair, with your feet four inches apart. With elbows out, grab both knees, holding on to the insides. Try to push your knees toward each other while pulling them apart with your arms. Hold for a count of ten. Rest ten or twenty seconds and try again. This fine isometric tightens loose muscle on the inside of the thighs through dynamic tension, but you *must* do it every day. It's a good arm tightener too.

For getting rid of sagging, crepey skin: Here's an exception to doing exercise on the bed. If you're not going to a gym, lie face

down on the bed, legs together; raise one leg at a time slowly, from knee to toe, to a position approximately eight inches above the bed. Your thighs don't move. Now place one foot against the heel of your other foot. Apply pressure at heels, forcing one against the other. Now reverse. This isometric or dynamic-tension exercise strengthens the hamstring area and tightens muscles at the back of the thighs.

Crinkled, crepey or mottled skin at the back of the thighs comes to many women in their middle years. This particular exercise gets that skin in shape for shorts or bathing suit. (For a good, complementary exercise for backs of legs and buttocks, try Step 4 on p. 49.)

Most experts agree the most difficult part of the body to exercise is the buttocks, although the largest human muscle of all, the gluteus maximus, is located there. You can feel it when you're sitting. The best way to **reduce the size of buttocks** is to duck walk, or walk in a squatting position. You also build up the gluteus maximus, displacing fat with solid tissue. Maybe it won't bring weight reduction, but it *will* help get rid of the added inches. That's what is important.

Another, easier exercise for the buttocks is alternately tightening and flexing the gluteus maximus muscle thirty times. Rest briefly and repeat twice, for a total of ninety. This exercise, again, must be practiced daily if it is to be effective.

It may seem a bit overpowering at the beginning, but once these exercises become routine, they shouldn't take up more than twenty minutes a day. They may be the most important time of day, a real investment in good health and beauty.

There are other exercises, of course. No exercise is really bad, but I find calisthenics the very best exercise program of all. They can—indeed, they *must*—be practiced every day without fail. Many women chart an exercise program for themselves and pursue it enthusiastically for a few days or weeks, then begin to skip a day here and there; pretty soon they forget about it entirely. It would be better not to start at all; such defeat is chalked up psychologically as another failure.

Here are some tips for making exercise more effective:

1   Don't engage in calisthenics or sports right after eating. Try to wait at least two hours before exerting yourself. Exercise on a full stomach is quickly exhausting, and can lead to sickness or dizziness.

2   Once a calisthenics schedule is a regular part of your life, branch out by taking up tennis, swiming, golf, or some other sport that can become a part of your social life. You'll be surprised how much your stamina has improved through those daily exercises.

3   If necessary, join a gym or health club. Many women will stay with an exercise program only if there are others on the same daily regimen. It's more fun with other people, too!

4   Bathe after you work out; it's refreshing and stimulating. Or shower; the water washes away perspiration and leaves you tingling.

And remind yourself that whatever you're doing, you'll do it better if you're feeling good and looking good. By shaping up, you feel better to yourself and to others, inside and out.

6

Eating Is Controlled Cheating

In our culture it's a sin, if not a crime, to be fat. It's supposedly best to have the lean, sleek look of semistarvation. No matter how beautiful the face, how porcelain the skin, how lovely the nature and soul of a woman, if she is overweight she can't honestly accept herself as attractive. And nobody else can, either!

In other, heftier fashion eras, extra padding was an asset. Ancient Greek and Roman women were delightfully plump. The stunning women of Rubens's era couldn't have weighed in at an ounce less than one hundred and eighty pounds each, nude.

In twentieth-century Europe and America, our model is Twiggy. Well, almost. For better or for worse, thanks to couturiers and Madison Avenue (and, yes, movies and television), men and women are now doomed to look as if we'd just survived famine. Barely.

How do we get that way? *Diet*, of course!

As a woman I've always been intimidated by magazine advertising. The chic models seem as thin as the pencil I nervously chew while I'm looking at them. At fashions shows I've felt like a cow because the mannequins were wearing size five or less.

Foundation garments, corsets, and girdles have all but disappeared, thank God, but at what cost to women? It's no use trying to hide or disguise that excess weight on our frames; it has to be removed—for good.

Exercise has relatively little effect on weight loss. Even run-

56

And here's what the movies did to me

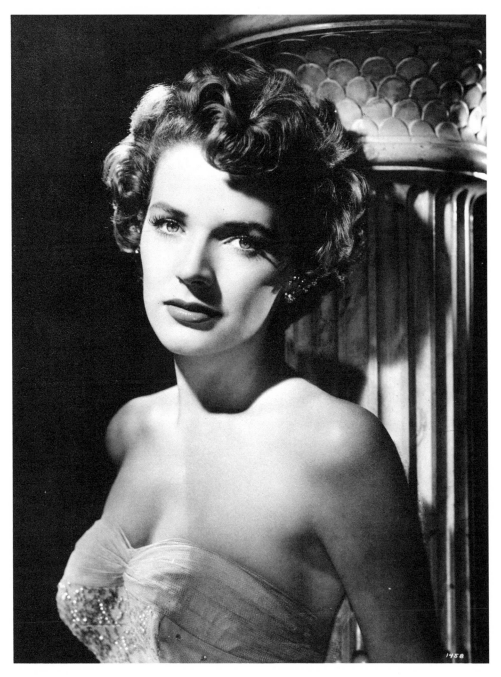

So now I was becoming a movie star, but what those studios did with my identity I wouldn't wish on a juggler. This is my Deborah Kerr phase.

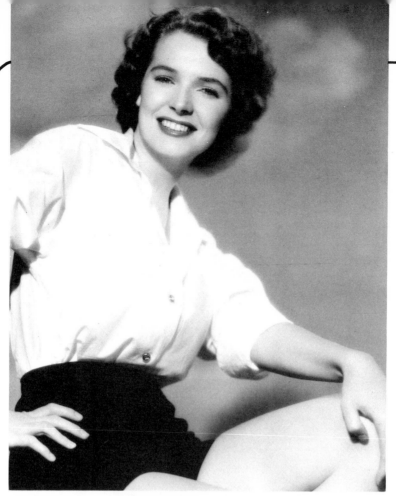

Here I am at Paramou
the wholesome, outdoor
type at 18 (left)
and virginal even as
a sweater girl (bottom

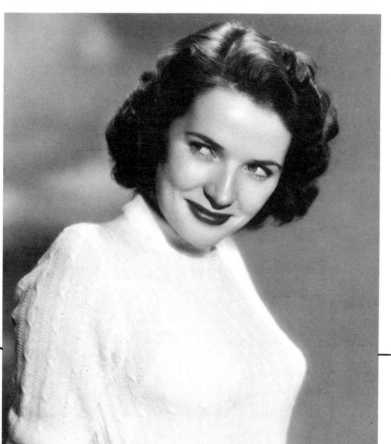

At Metro (right) I was
but they dressed me
like a 35-year-old.
The movie was Half A
Hero with Red Skelton.

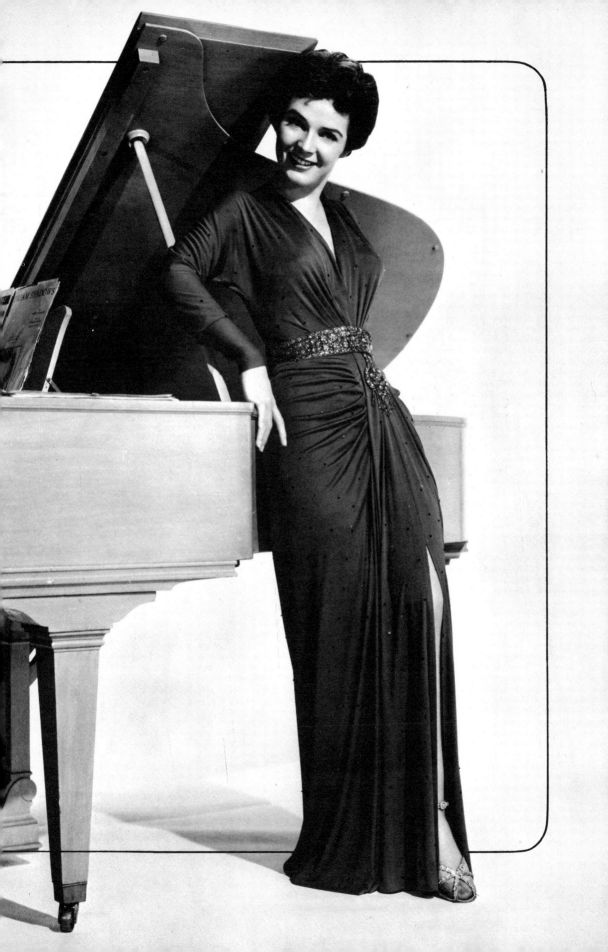

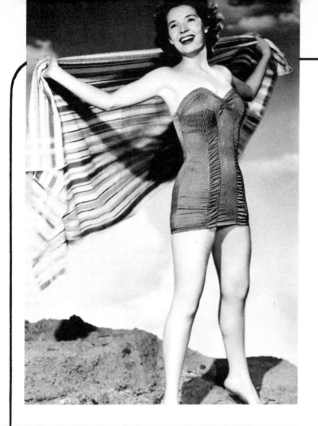

Identity, identity. Everybody is supposed to one. Right? Well, I had dozens, but unfortun none of them was really me—certainly not in show business years. They made me a sire songbird. A young matron. They put me bathing suit with my bulgy thighs; holy smoke, didn't I have sense enough at least to stay out of one? But the picture (top right) on the right-page is a milestone. I was at the peak of my ca singing at the Riviera Hotel in Las Vegas. Su right? Sure, but who was I?

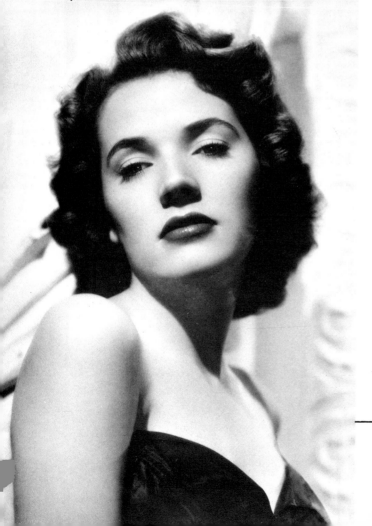

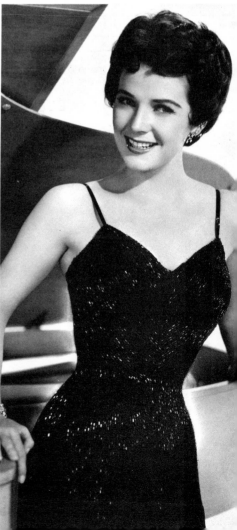

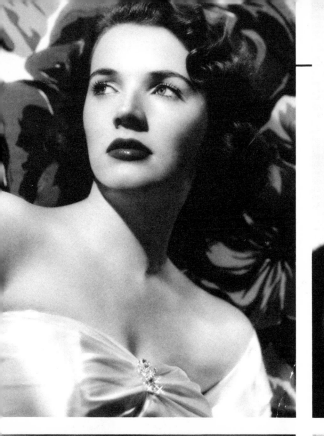

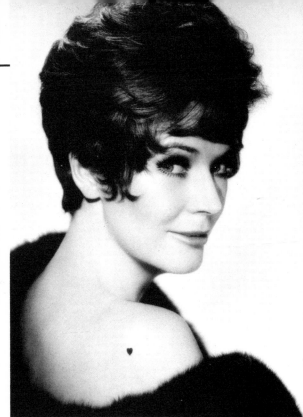

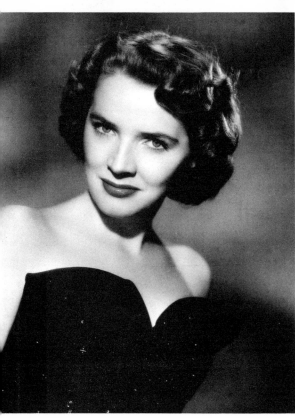

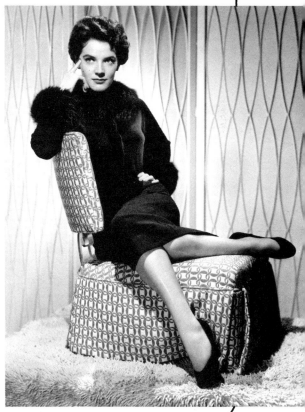

So eventually I got sexy

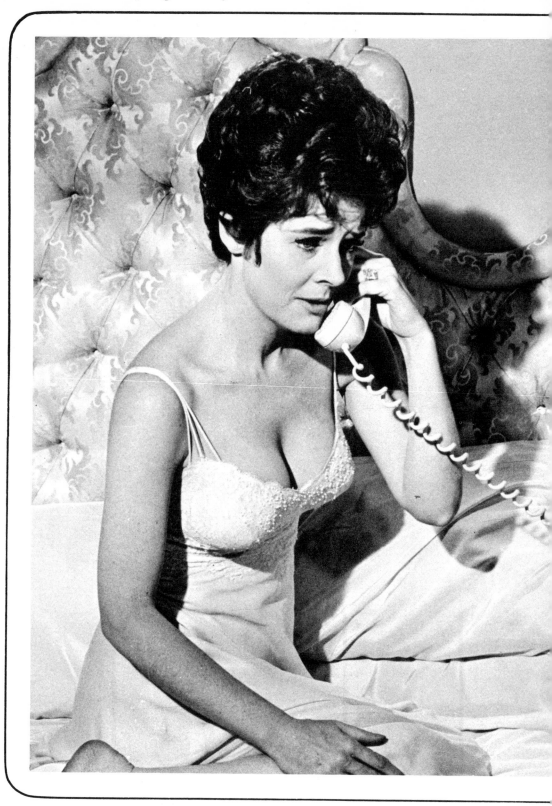

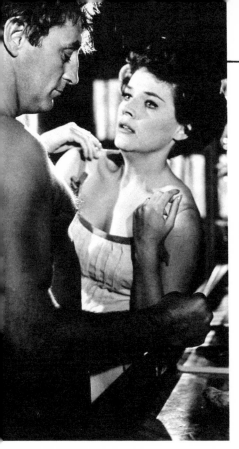

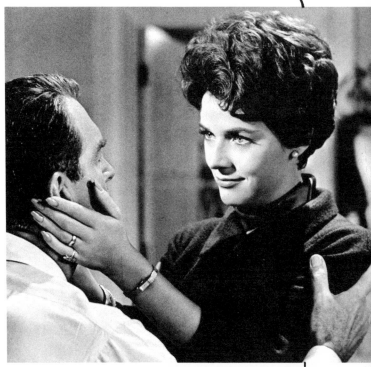

a dumb dingbat in Move Over, Darling (opposite). *Got by Robert Mitchum in Cape Fear (above, left). I was elected* st woman president (with Fred MacMurray as my consort) in s for My President (top right and bottom), *and resigned* se of "pregnancy" (right). *I won no Oscars, but I had fun.*

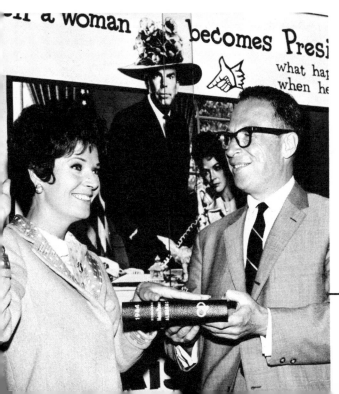

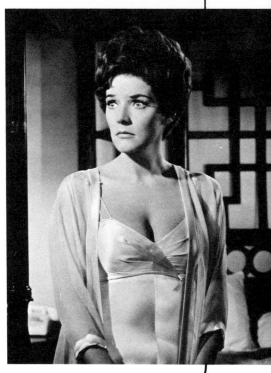

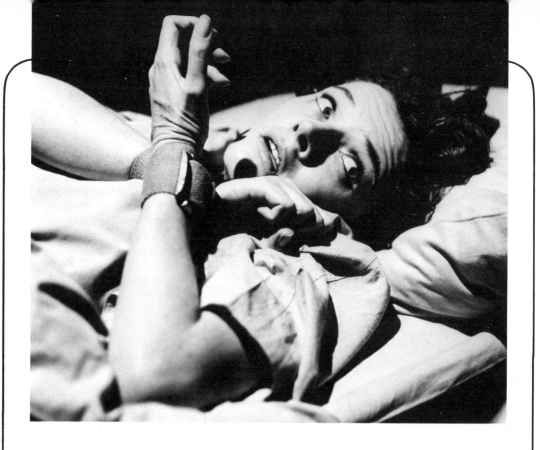

In The Caretakers *I had to become a mental patient—and a real actress. It was rough on me—so rough that I went into real-life therapy just as soon as the picture was finished.*

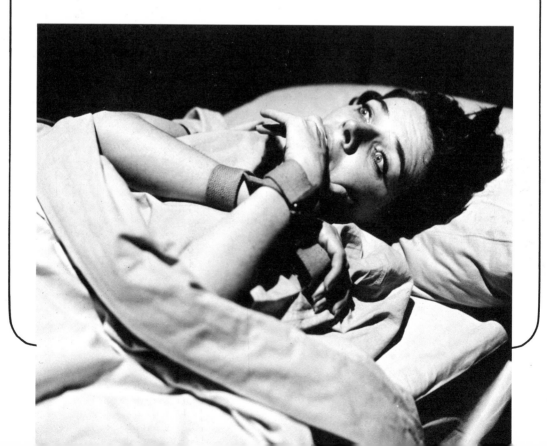

ning two miles full tilt burns off only a handful of calories. Good for firming up the body? Yes. For reducing weight? No.

Fat men have grown rich writing books telling women how to become thin. I know; I've tried almost every diet in the past twenty years, from *The Drinking Man's Diet* to *Dr. Atkins' Diet Revolution*. And all those in between. And then I've read criticisms of these diets by equally fat male doctors.

The din of would-be authorities in the diet field confirms me more and more in my violent opposition to fad diets. For that's what they are. My strong reaction has nothing to do with how well or how badly the individual diet works. The point is, no man or woman can spend the rest of his or her life eating fish, fowl, and cottage cheese and drinking eight glasses of water, or whatever the fad diet recommends.

There comes a time when every human being has that overwhelming desire to eat a rich vegetable, creamy salad, a dessert, a piece of candy or fruit, and maybe he wants beer or wine, or a healthy shot of booze.

I've never known a professional dietitian who could assure me or anyone else that a particular diet—aside from those administered by doctors in critical areas of health—could be tolerated by our bodies year in and year out.

I have my own diet, one I can live with. I've managed to stay on it for more than five years. Though it's essentially a maintaining diet, it will help you lose weight if you're simply overweight. If you're obese, you need medical advice. And don't hesitate. Chronic overweight can be a sign of psychological problems. You should discuss any serious weight problems with your doctor— with your own personal physician, who knows you. *Never* a diet doctor.

Weight Watchers is a good way to lose weight, and many of my friends have been successful Weight Watchers. But no diet in the world can stop the cravings for particular foods that come up now and then, even in people who aren't the least bit pregnant.

So people are going to cheat. That's human nature. And when they do, the weight comes back, with only stretch marks and flabby skin to show it ever went away.

I have a built-in cheating system in my diet. I guess if it were a commercial program for weight loss, it might be called "The Cheater's Diet." (I'll explain the cheating later.)

The *first* step in my diet is to eliminate temptation as much as possible. Everybody gets hungry, and I'm no different. So I get rid of all the candy and peanuts in the house. If it's there, I know I'll grab it.

Instead I have little containers of carrots, celery, radishes, and cherry tomatoes on the cocktail table, or around my desk or make-up table. Sometimes cheese, but in thin sticks. If I feel the need to snack I can, without adding a lot of useless calories, and these foods are nourishing.

The *second* step is to convince myself it's possible to enjoy my life and diet, and that I'm controlling my shape as much as I am my weight. The fact is, shape is more important than weight in any diet; it's what your body *looks* like that's important, after all, and exercise in conjunction with diet is absolutely necessary. As the weight comes off, the skin and muscles must be kept in tone to take up the slack left by the departing fat. It's possible for a woman to be the perfect weight for her height, yet still have an abominable figure.

I fluctuate between perfect weight and bad figure, and imperfect weight and good figure. I've had a near perfect figure when my weight was many pounds over what I would have liked it to be.

Weight charts are meaningless. They often indicate you could be much heavier or lighter than you are, because they pay no attention to bone structure and weight distribution. What if you have the bone structure of a canary? Suppose you have the solid frame of a Green Bay Packers's tackle? The ideal weight on the average doctor's wall chart is about a ton heavier—give or take a few pounds—than the average woman would like to be. The chart assumes that the woman reading it is a perfect physical specimen, ready to enter eight events in the Olympic Games.

Two women can be five feet six inches and weigh one hundred and twenty-five pounds. Each has her weight distributed differently than the other. One has a great figure; the other looks ghastly.

Bone structure is all-important. I weigh one hundred and twenty-two pounds. Usually people guess that I weigh ten pounds less. I can make a bundle from Guess-Your-Weight people at country fairs. What helps to give the illusion of slenderness is my broad shoulders—bone structure. The shoulders are so broad that everything below them looks skinny. On the other hand, very narrow shoulders tend to make women with normal hips look broad and hippy. It's all a matter of proportion.

So my diet is tuned in to this type of body. However, the diet is *equally* effective for any woman (or man) without specific medical problems relating to weight contol.

It isn't a starvation diet; it fills me up and keeps me content between meals. When I was on those crazy quick diets I felt starved all the time and kept on reaching for anything edible. Not any more. I realized I can't live without vegetables, salads, fruit, and an occasional sweet. *So I cheat.*

The basis of my diet is convincing myself that my eyes are smaller than my stomach. When I was little, my mother told me to eat everything on my plate: "Think of the poor starving children in China." At the time I wasn't sensible enough to reason that one out, asking myself what eating all the food in front of me had to do with some poor kid in China, so I ate everything on my plate. And to this day I eat everything that's put in front of me. That's why I have to *control what's put there in the first place.*

I gave up eating in cafeterias because whenever I'm in one, I have a compelling desire to eat the steam tables empty. There's nothing I can pass up. So I got my eyes used to seeing less food on the plate. It sets me up psychologically: Seeing less is, hopefully, wanting less.

First Week:

> I eat exactly as I have done all my life, including such fattening foods as bread, butter, sweets, potatoes, and the rest; *but* I cut the portions in half. *Exactly in half.* If I usually had two tablespoons of mashed potatoes and gravy, I take a single tablespoon. If dinner includes a whole steak, I eat half a steak. Instead of two eggs for breakfast, I have one. I eat a small piece of cherry pie instead of a large one.
>
> At the end of a week, my eyes are used to seeing *half* as much as they saw before. And that half becomes my normal portion. The helpings seem generous enough after only a single week.

Second Week:

> Now I remove everything that's super-fattening from my diet: bread, butter, potatoes, desserts, etc. But I *double* the portions of

the rest of my meal: meat, eggs, cheese, vegetables, fruit—the satisfying things.

Wow! I look at the plate and all the food is overwhelming! The helpings are twice the size I've become used to during the first week of the diet. Psychologically it doesn't feel as if I'm on a diet at all. I eat a whole steak, two tablespoons of green beans instead of one. A full diet in place of half a diet.

Third Week:

Now it's time to start on the normal routine, *my lifetime diet.* I measure my food at between one-half and three-quarters of a portion.

For breakfast I allow myself a slice of toast with my eggs. Already I'm controlling my cheating. Instead of eliminating bread altogether, I have one slice with breakfast. Maybe every third or fourth day I'll have a dessert that I shouldn't have. I try to eat just half of it, because I know that makes me feel incredibly good, *but I will have cheated.* And that's OK, because I know it. I'm not kidding myself.

I'm happy with keeping my weight more or less even. If I discover I've gained a little, then I cut back on quantities. I'm my own diet authority. I can cheat. I have dressing on my salad (though not blue cheese or a heavy cream dressing). I don't eliminate salt or sugar. I don't totally banish butter from my toast. I can afford to have dessert twice a week or so because I watch the portions.

Of course, there are lapses, and holidays occur. When my weight really goes up, I start on the **First Week** schedule and follow through the **Third Week** steps until my weight is back at one hundred twenty-two pounds.

Common sense is very much part of the diet. Rich, heavy foods should always be avoided, since they're fattening even in small amounts. But if I have an overwhelming need for a fancy pastry now and then, I put it under the heading of *Cheating;* I have it and enjoy it. I realize, though, that I'll have to compensate by going without regular helpings of other foods at the next meal.

I try to avoid set patterns in meals. I like as much variation in breakfast, lunch, and dinner as possible.

But *breakfast* is typically eggs. Though I'll have three from time to time, my usual maximum is two. I have them boiled, fried, scrambled, coddled, or poached—it doesn't matter, so long as they're not the same every day. I have two very crisp strips of bacon with either an English muffin or a piece of toast.

If I discover I've put on a pound and a half, say, the day before, I cut down to one egg and a piece of toast—no bacon. This is my built-in *cheating-compensation system.*

I don't have orange juice for breakfast, ever. It was the first thing to come out of my diet, because of its enormous sugar content. Instead I drink grapefruit, tomato, prune, or V-8 juice.

Skim milk turns me off, so I drink whole milk. I use artificial sweeteners whenever I can. If I have cereal, every once in a while, I use whole milk. And once every two months or so I'll go absolutely wild on French toast or pancakes for breakfast. Next morning I weigh myself and immediately go back to half portions.

At midday I try to eat lightly, because I enjoy breakfast and dinner more than lunch. Why not emphasize the positive aspects of dieting by fully enjoying two meals and letting the third one slide a bit? Doctors say, and I agree, that a hearty breakfast is the most important meal of the day. That doesn't mean you have to stuff yourself like a goose, but it makes more sense to eat a lot in the morning than to glut yourself at noon and spend the rest of the day half asleep, or devour a huge dinner and lie awake half the night trying to digest it.

A typical *lunch* for me is cold cuts or cheese or cottage cheese—maybe some of each. I'll have pickles and olives too. Bland food bores me. Everything's more interesting when it's a little spicy.

Dinner's often a salad and steak or fish. It could be stew or hamburgers. Spaghetti once in a while, and that dessert maybe twice a week.

That's it. For the social drinking most of us do, my diet rules still apply: Cut the wine or liquor consumption in half. I happen to prefer wine to hard liquor. I especially like white wine, and often have it on the rocks instead of a highball. If you like liquor, have it straight. Mixed drinks add calories and fluid. A straight whiskey will get you where you want to be as quickly as a Manhattan, and you'll be thinner when you get there. (Of course, if you have drinking problems, that's another story, and you probably won't be too concerned about a diet anyway.)

A major factor in dieting is the psychological ability to diet without surrendering a particular category of foods—sweets, starches, liquor—for the rest of your life.

Diet is an integral part of beauty. Proper weight, good health, and eight hours' sleep a night are the basic ingredients for attractiveness. But they must come naturally, without any "magic" potions, like diet pills or sleeping pills.

Diet pills are an artificial way of reducing and end up being a crutch, or worse. They lead you to believe you can't lose weight without pills, and who wants to live with weight-reducing pills forever? Most of them are based on amphetamines, or "speed," an unnatural upper, sometimes addictive, and you probably know that you quickly build up resistance to them, so they become worthless as appetite depressants.

To diet with pills is to risk your health. The emotional side effects of crash diets are devastating enough because of the radical reduction in food intake. No reasonable person needs the added hypertension of amphetamines.

Also, some dermatologists have proven that crash diets accompanied by amphetamines do hideous things to the skin. Sudden and dramatic weight loss, especially if you omit toning exercises, leaves stretch marks, or results in crepey, hanging skin. And that's just another problem you don't need.

Many, many movie stars, naked and without plastic surgery, are dreadful examples of what crash diets and pills can do. They are victims of the screen, too fat to play roles at their natural weights. They go on suicidal diets to lose twenty or thirty pounds for a picture in a couple of weeks' time. In addition to destroying their skin, the emotional costs are substantial.

Those stars who can't force themselves to diet are treated by doctors with special injections. It's all very hush-hush, and probably should be. Common sense tells me that if this were approved by the American Medical Association, we would be better informed on serums to decrease weight. I've seen some of my movie-star friends lose dramatic amounts of weight through injections, but they're also on pills. The results aren't all in yet, but from where I stand I'm not sure I wouldn't prefer being overweight to being dependent on speed or a hypodermic needle.

Parents who worry about their children getting involved with drugs should check their own medicine cabinets. Between the diet pills, the tranquilizers, and the sleeping pills, they probably have enough for a Sweet Sixteen drug party. And another thing parents should remember is not to overfeed their children. Eating habits are developed in the first months of life. The sweet, plump baby will become a plump and probably unhappy teenager.

Eating is a lifetime occupation that you start the day you're born. It's a great pleasure. But if you want a good figure, you have to learn controlled cheating when you're eating. That way you can have your cake *and* eat it!

7

Face Up

The best beauty treatment for your skin is to fall in love, stay in love, or find a new love. Everything feels and looks better. That gives an outer glow to your skin. Your skin becomes more supple when you're in love. There's a brightness in your smile. Eyes shine.

Fabergé and The Polly Bergen Company can't bottle love. And neither, I feel safe in saying, can any of our competitors. The next best thing is learning to treat our faces lovingly. And that means, first of all, cleanliness. It doesn't matter how many moisturizers or night creams or make-up products are used; if your face isn't clean to begin with, you're in trouble.

Make-up is secondary. First you must have a healthy skin, and that means a clean skin. For most of my life I washed my face with soap and water. That's what my mother used on her face, and so I followed her example. Though I began using a cleansing cream when I was in my thirties, I still feel physically unclean if I don't use soap and water. So I compromise: cleanser at night, water in the morning.

The earlier a girl begins taking care of her skin, the better. I introduced Kathy and P.K. to skin cleansers before they were in their teens. Like me, like my daughters, most girls imitate their mothers in grooming. I didn't know what kind of animal a dermatologist was until I was in my twenties, but my girls have regular appointments with one. They're both very aware of skin care. P.K. has thin, dry skin. She began using a moisturizer when she was twelve. Kathy has dark, oily skin and has been using a deep-pore cleanser (a mild abrasive) since she was eleven. I'm certain they'll both have better skin at my age than I do, because they learned to take care of them before any damage was done.

Two cardinal rules should be followed by all women. I wish I could get them passed by Congress, or at least the state legislatures.

Number one: Any woman who doesn't use a moisturizer is committing facial suicide. This includes women with oily skin. There's a difference between oil and moisture, and any woman who wears make-up without first applying moisturizer is doing to herself what her worst enemy couldn't do to her.

Number two: Never, never go to bed with your make-up on. Of course, if you're not too sure of the man you're sleeping with, the early-morning shock of your naked face may be too much for his sensitive soul, and away he goes. In that case, break the truth to him gradually, removing elements of your make-up a little at a time. But if make-up stays on the skin too long, it will certainly damage it.

Caring for skin is easy. Here's what I do and, with variations for skin type, I'm sure it's a sound program for all women.

Step 1: I remove my make-up every night with cleansing foam. Foam doesn't run as easily as lotion or cream, and so it doesn't irritate my eyes. The foam disintegrates immediately, getting into the skin and starting the dirt and bacteria moving. Women who prefer the texture of cream or lotion should use that. (My line includes all three forms.)

I move the foam up and out with my hands, without pushing the skin. Then I start removing it with white cotton balls. White —that's how you can tell when your face is clean. No decorator colors. If you have an uncontrollable urge to get pink, yellow, blue, or aquamarine cotton balls, put them in your guest room. Let your guests worry about their skin; you're going to use white.

Step 2: After removing that first layer of cleanser, I saturate the cotton ball with freshener. (Oily-skinned women would use the deep-pore astringent to control excess oil.) I go over my face gently and look at the cotton. It's filthy. I throw it away, get another, and repeat until I have a clean, clean white cotton ball in my hand—maybe the eighth or tenth.

The *most important* step in cleaning the face is not the cleanser, it's the rinser (another name for freshener). Women with very dry skins may be tempted not to use a rinser, because they think it's very drying and will leave a parched feeling. But that's not so. Every woman must take the second step.. The rinser makes the difference between clean and not clean. To use a cleanser and not follow up with a rinser is just like washing your face with soap and wiping it off on a towel.

Also: Never use tissues. They have wood-fiber content which can be very destructive to the skin. Use only cotton, in some form.

Step 3: Now I've removed all my make-up and I'm ready for night treatment. I use my Night Concentrate very thinly over the *entire* face, with a little extra in the real disaster areas: the eyes, mouth, and neck. Just that, and I'm ready for bed.

All of us in the cosmetics business naturally want to sell as many products as possible. So a woman goes to a cosmetics counter and says she wants something for the night. "Terrific," says the salesperson. "Now, here's something for your eyes. This for your throat. A new product for your left nostril. This here goes on your forehead, and our new cheek cream for left and right cheeks." The woman goes home laden with jars; if she's like me, she puts the throat cream on the eyes, the forehead one on the nose, and eventually gets so disgusted she throws all of them away and doesn't even bother. Or she faithfully applies half a dozen products at night, and by the time she comes to bed her man's in his second sleep cycle.

So I created Night Concentrate, and I've found that's all I need. I put it on the lines I'm beginning to discover on my neck, I put it wherever it's needed, and I use it to prevent future disaster areas.

I've cleaned, rinsed, put the night treatment on. Now I try for my eight hours' sleep. I rarely succeed, but that's what I try to get. When I wake up my skin feels slightly moist and fresh. There's nothing sticky or greasy about the night treatment, nothing to turn off the man at your side. It doesn't discolor the pillowcase or get into your hair—or his.

Step 4: In the morning, I wash my face. Many women don't bother to clean their faces again in the morning if they did it at night, rationalizing that they've gone nowhere to get their faces dirty. So they start out applying a moisturizer and foundation—ouch!

Dirt, grime, and bacteria are in the air all the time, and settle on the face during the night. Dirt tends to stick to moist skin, attracted by the night cream. So in the morning I use soap, because of my hangup about not feeling clean unless I've washed with soap and water. But my soap is super-fatted and oil-based, with almost the consistency of a cream. It *doesn't* dry out the skin. I build up a lather on my hands and lightly massage my face. Then I rinse with lukewarm water, as should all women with dry skin. Hot water draws oil to the surface and flushes it away—which is fine for oily skins.

While washing, I'm careful not to push or stretch my skin. Then I go through the rinsing process, this time with water, never less than fifteen times. I never use a face cloth. It's too harsh; its texture just encourages burst capillaries in skin like mine.

Then I *pat* my face dry. The softer and more absorbent the towel the better, but I never rub. Rubbing the skin—on face or body—stretches the surface skin.

Step 5: After washing and drying, I apply probably the most important cosmetic product of all: moisturizer. A good moisturizer does more for your skin than any other preparation, and for many a young woman that's all she needs. It replenishes natural moisture removed through washing, perspiration, or evaporation. Also, it leaves an occlusive film that seals the moisture into the face and also creates a barrier for the pores, as though "waterproofing" the skin against dirt.

My best gauge for measuring the effectiveness of a particular moisturizer is comparing it to Chinese food: If your face is hungry for more more moisturizer two hours after you've applied it, then it isn't doing the job.

Most of us tend to think of ourselves as oily- or dry-skinned; that's not quite accurate. Almost all women have some facial areas that are oily, some dry, and some that seem perfectly balanced between the two. Like most others, I describe my complexion by the area that seems dominant, and most of my face is dry. But there are oily places around the nose, in that T-zone on the forehead between the eyes, and around my chin. On the other hand, there's exteme dryness around my eyes and cheeks. A moisturizer evens up the distribution of natural skin moisture, equalizes the oily and dry patches, and prevents make-up from shifting.

Otherwise, the make-up runs on the oily surfaces and flakes on the dry. As the day wears on, these differences become more noticeable and you end up with a streaked look on your face, which is total disaster.

I usually put on make-up at seven or seven thirty in the morning, and don't reapply it for the rest of the day, except to powder my nose if it gets shiny or put on more lipstick after I've chewed it off. This is possible through my moisturizer. Before I used it my make-up "slid" around and my skin felt like an alligator's. I looked like I had a communicable disease, with the little dry flakes on my face.

Basically, *a skin needs moisturizing, cleansing, rinsing, and night treatment every day to keep healthy and glowing.* But there are individual skin problems, most with solutions. I live and work in two cities (Los Angeles and New York) and am a victim of city air. (You know, the kind you can see.) So I have clogged pores, and I use a deep-pore cleanser three times a week to slough off the dead skin. I don't use it daily; even though it's gentle, the product is, after all, an abrasive.

My deep-pore cleanser is called Scrub and is made of crushed almonds, essential oils, honey, and other absorbing ingredients to pull oil out of the pores. It smells like marzipan and is deep apricot in color. I use it on my freshly cleaned and damp face, around the nose, chin, and between the eyes, massaging gently to open the pores without stretching the skin. Then I rinse with lukewarm water followed by freshener. Both my rinses contain allantoin, an anti-bacterial agent. The rinser closes the pores again while acting as an antiseptic.

This procedure is good for all pore problems: blackheads, whiteheads, pimples, and such. If you scream at your daughter for not cleaning her face properly, you might be underestimating the problem. Using soap or a cleanser might not be enough; the trouble starts lower down, and the outer layer of skin must be removed.

Tightening up the skin is something else again, and I don't

approve of it. I don't have a mask in my line and won't have one. The term "mask" comes from the ancient facial masks that were actually fitted to the contours of the face. Now, of course, it refers to a solution which tightens the skin when applied to the face. It can give a minor face lift for two or three hours, until the face drops again. Ultimately it stretches the skin. Common sense tells you that. If something makes the skin taut and releases it after a couple of hours, it must stretch skin if used over a period of time. But I suppose anything's possible, and if the day ever comes when a mask is developed that isn't injurious, I'll be the first to market it.

But I don't believe in miracles. I wasn't brought up that way. Even if there *were* miracles, they wouldn't come in jars. So, to the claim "Buy this cream and it will make your wrinkles disappear," I say: "No way, José!"

There are no wrinkle removers except for plastic surgeons. Creams can soften wrinkles, deemphasize lines, maybe even help puff up little ones that are just starting, but they can't remove them.

There's one simple test for all cosmetic claims: Does it work? And does it work on me? Women should test products themselves. It it doesn't work for you, forget that it's the favorite of movie stars, Mrs. Onassis, or the Queen of England. And if it *does* work for you, stay with it. Your beauty routine will be more effective and efficient. And learn how to apply the product. Even the best cleanser or moisturizer won't do you much good if you stretch your skin whenever you put it on.

Be gentle with your face. The older you get, the more your skin loses its elasticity. Young girls get rid of fatigue lines by going to bed early. When you're older, that's not enough. But loss of elasticity isn't the aging process alone—we carelessly and possibly purposely abuse our facial skin.

The less you move your skin, the longer it will retain elasticity. Never massage your face inward—that creates lines. Stroke your face; treat it lovingly, gently. Facials are bad if the person giving them pulls and tugs the skin like rubber. Facial exercises are as bad or worse. Chronic animation can stretch skin, and that's one of my problems. I'm *too* animated; I use every muscle in my face to express myself. That doesn't mean I should become deadpan or look like a corpse, but I never move my face around when I'm washing or cleaning.

So forget facial movement and work with creams, or love. Creams *and* love are best. But if you're waiting for that love, or in between loves, or it's not yet rekindled, learn to treat your face as though you love it. If your face shows signs of being loved, chances are it will be.

8

Protect Your Own Hide

Before we consider the rest of your skin—that gorgeous covering over all of you—here are some basic do's and don't's for skin care.

- DO USE THE PROPER BASE FOUNDATION FOR YOUR TYPE SKIN.
- DO KEEP THE SKIN CLEAN.
- DO USE AMPLE BATH OILS.
- DO FIGHT TENSION AND STRESS.
- DO WORK WITH CREAMS RATHER THAN SOAP AND WATER IN COLD WEATHER.
- DO RINSE YOUR FACE THOROUGHLY EVERY TIME YOU APPLY CREAM.
- DO CARRY AN EMOLLIENT STICK TO MOISTURIZE AROUND THE EYES.
- DO VISIT A DERMATOLOGIST AS YOU WOULD A GYNECOLOGIST.
- DO PAY THE SAME ATTENTION TO YOUR BODY AS YOU WOULD YOUR FACE.
- DO DRINK A LOT OF WATER.

On the negative side:

- DON'T PRACTICE FACIAL EXERCISES.
- DON'T USE TOO MUCH HEAVY FOUNDATION MAKE-UP.
- DON'T HAVE FACIAL MASSAGE.
- DON'T EXPOSE YOUR SKIN TO TOO MUCH SUN.
- DON'T GET TOO LITTLE SLEEP.
- DON'T EAT IMPROPERLY.

71

- DON'T USE STRONG ABRASIVES.
- DON'T USE HORMONE CREAMS (THEY ENCOURAGE HAIR GROWTH).
- DON'T EXPOSE YOURSELF TO STEAM HEAT OR TOO MUCH AIR CONDITIONING.
- DON'T USE TIGHTENING FACE MASKS.

And the most important rule of all is: *Stop smoking,* or never start. Cigarette smoke is the most destructive element in modern life, aside from the sun. I'm an authority on both—I've tanned my skin to near-destruction and I've smoked my entire adult life, paying the price with clogged pores, lack of good circulation, and skin discolored to nicotinic yellow. But I go on smoking, hoping for the strength to quit one day.

Three times in my life I've tried to stop smoking. But I'm super-tense, almost hyperkinetic, with more energy than a hothouse full of hummingbirds. I've convinced myself that cigarette smoking keeps me on the ground. I think of it as a weight I wear to prevent me from flying off into the stratosphere. Those times I tried to quit turned me into a basket case. My children became basket cases, my husband threatened to leave me (he ultimately did anyway), and I began puffing away again.

On an emotional basis, I don't really want to quit. Cary Grant once sent me to a hypnotist to help me break the habit. It didn't work. Cary is one of those obnoxious converts. *He* stopped smoking, and makes life unbearable for anyone who hasn't. He won't even light my cigarettes, and if I'm out of matches I could die before he'd find one for me—and even then he wouldn't.

Smoking creates facial wrinkles. It's deeply injurious not only to the lungs, but to the heart, skin, eyes—even to fingernails, hair, and teeth. As a beauty deterrent, it is unsurpassed. And so, gentle reader, in the best tradition of do-as-I-say-not-as-I-do, I tell you: *Stop smoking now!* And to the nonsmoker: *Don't ever start!*

I'm also an authority on ravages of the sun. When I first returned from New York to California in 1961, I had a pure peaches-and-cream white skin. There wasn't a mark anywhere on my body or face. A few freckles sprinkled around my nose from childhood, but otherwise not a mark, not a mole, not a line, not a single burst capillary. Nothing—just pure white skin.

I managed to survive that way in Hollywood for three years. Then I became embarrassed at being a mobile alabaster statue every summer while all the other women I knew were toasted golden brown. Freddie and I took a house at Malibu, and I decided to join the "sun-and-more-sun" set—I didn't know any better.

In those three summer months I got the first suntan of my life. I *really* got it. I burned and peeled and burned and peeled. But I worked on. A lot of women will remember the process, and it's not much fun. Stretched out for hours in the sun, squinting to read a book (and bringing all those little lines hurrying around your eyes), listening to the radio, trying to doze—it's like sitting under a dryer or being stretched out on a drying rack. Sun bathing is usually a chore and a bore, a so-called beauty treatment. But who enjoys perspiring, batting at sand flies, or sitting like a cake in the oven, waiting to turn golden?

I didn't. But I finally had my tan. Hallelujah! My skin changed forever. After that summer it never returned to its peaches-and-cream self. And I've had to learn to live with burst capillaries. My skin is very thin and the blood lies close to the surface.

These tiny little red marks can be removed if you catch them early enough. But once the little radiations begin to spread, it's almost impossible to remove the burst capillary altogether. An electric needle will remove them early on, and I have them burned off such obvious places as the end of my nose. But if they're neglected too long, they require surgery.

Burst capillaries is *one* reason for not exposing yourself to lots of sun; drying out and aging the skin is *another*, though the best reason for not broiling yourself to a desirable nut color in that sunbathing increases the incidence of skin cancer. Some sunshine is good for everybody, but the amount of exposure depends on a woman's skin type. A little sunshine in your life brings Vitamin C and chases away that pasty-faced look. On excessively oily skin, the sun's rays can even be helpful, by drying up excess oils and speeding natural body secretion.

But overexposure is probably the single most destructive thing a woman can do to her skin, particularly if it's very dry or sensitive. The natural blond with deep brown summer skin is virtually tanning her own hide. Furriers tan hides by stretching out the skin and drying it. That makes leather, and that's what people do to themselves. They age themselves incredibly, and it's immediately noticeable. Old skin means an old woman. Young skin, young girl.

Sunshine actually changes the molecular structure of the skin, and it's only a matter of time before the skin stretches. First you have tiny networks of fine lines at the pucker areas of the face: the corners of eyes and mouth, on the forehead, and around the neck. Then the skin begins to sag and dry out, aging a woman far beyond her years.

I now do my damndest to minimize the rigors of sun and the other elements. I try to avoid extremes of temperature and climate, and I use creams. Though no cream can stop the aging process, much less reverse it, a good cream can slow the process even for those women who think the boat has already sailed, possibly with their own skins as sails.

In the summer, I rinse off in fresh water when I get out of the ocean. Salt crusts on the skin; it's drying and gritty and uncomfortable. Even when I'm out in the wilderness on rugged vacations (I love them), I care for my skin, consider its needs.

Last summer I took a raft trip down the Colorado River with P.K. and Peter. We slept in sleeping bags in the open, and when it rained, it rained on us—we didn't even have a tent. I washed in the river, almost drowned about twenty times, and lost sixteen tubes of soap in the current. (I use tubes with bio-degradable soap because I don't believe in ruining nature.) And in seven days I used two eight-ounce bottles of Hand and Body Moisturizer.

A woman should keep her skin moist and supple no matter where she is. At home, the bath is the best place for daily body care. I always bathe, never shower. Showers are more drying—fine for the woman with overall oily skin. When you use bath oil, it's almost impossible to dilute it and put it on your body after a shower.

The bath is also a great moment in the day, a time for luxury and relaxation, a time to pull yourself together. For oily skin, you can use Foaming Milk Bath, which softens the water (but doesn't add oils), makes bubbles, and is beautifully fragranced. I use it, but not alone, because my dry skin needs a body treatment in the tub. I use Deep Sea Bath Treatment, which adds oil to the water and acts as a moisturizer for my body. I step into the silky, milky bath and let everything float out of my mind. I forget the children, the business, the dinner menu; I'm relaxing in my own spa, and all women should take out five minutes a day for this.

I wash with superfatted soap which creams on the body. The

water is warm, not too hot (again, hot water is good for oily skins). My hair is brushed back off my face, and I've already put moisturizer on. With a nail brush, I push back the cuticles of my fingernails and toenails. I use a pumice stone on my feet.

When I come out of the bath, I *pat* myself dry and then rub my entire body down with Hand and Body Moisturizer. The light massage I give myself not only provides moisture, but gives me a nice sense of my body. I rub extra lotion on my legs and into my feet to prevent hard spots. In hot weather I add powder, spraying the mist all over me. It cools the body and the feet (I also spray my shoes). Women with oily skin can forget the body moisturizer and use only a talc or the Powder Mist Spray.

I bathe every night, for cleanliness and sensuality. It's a beautiful moment. In the morning, I wash my face and clean my ears, using Q-tips very cautiously. Ears are often forgotten. I find that a lot of wax collects in my ears, and every year or so I go deaf. Then I have them cleaned by a doctor. This is an area women should check out occasionally.

For personal cleanliness, I adore a bidet. It's the height of luxury. If you can't get one, remember a bath is better than a shower for personal hygiene. Douching can also be done, but remember: in moderation.

Clean skin is healthy skin, as I've said, but there can still be some beauty problems, like *body hair*. Some women aren't bothered by it. That's fine; they should leave it alone. But if hair on any part of your body becomes displeasing to you, get rid of it. Electrolysis is fine for hair on the breasts, stomach, or face. Oddly enough, on the body it's not at all painful. I had a few hairs removed electrolytically from my breasts and stomach. On the face it's something else. Electrolysis is sensational for removing moustaches, if you can handle it. I couldn't. You need the guts of a lion, but if you have them the results are fantastic. When I tried, I just went right off the chair. So I wax.

Some friends of mine are even strong enough to have electrolysis on and around the bikini line—a marvelous idea: You never have to worry about it again, and you don't have the ingrown-hair problem that comes from shaving. But I don't have that kind of courage. I shave.

For *legs* I recommend waxing. Of course, it's costly in both time and money. I have mine done, and it's expensive. I've also tried to do my own legs and ended up, a few hours later, with wax on the carpet, on the furniture, all over the place. It's a horror. If you can't have them waxed, shave your legs or use a depilatory. Shaving is very drying because it scrapes off the top layer of skin and tends to leave the legs flaky, so always use a lot of moisturizer. Use it excessively after shaving, and keep the legs well lubricated.

Underarms can be treated the same way as legs. I have many friends who wax, and that absolutely horrifies me. But then, leg waxing horrified me too in the beginning. My hardy friends usually start the underarm waxing in winter, when they really don't need to, so they can let the hair grow out a lot before waxing again. By the time they get to summer, when their underarms *are* exposed, they've really started to discourage the growth. They have it under control.

Eyebrows can be tweezed or waxed. Depilatories don't work, because you can't control them. For excessive facial down, waxing is the only solution. The down is blond, the hair follicles are extremely close together, and though it's not like dark facial hair, it picks up in the light and will be obvious under make-up. Waxing the hairline can pull the forehead up and bring out the eyes.

For very dark body hair, bleaching might be the answer. Though I know women who have their arms waxed, the totally hairless body isn't natural.

Discoloration of the skin (brown spots) can be caused by the sun, age, or hormones. Young girls on The Pill sometimes get terrible brown splotches on their bodies and faces. The Pill is a catalyst for these, and every woman should check with a dermatologist as well as her gynecologist or family doctor before taking it.

In fact, it's a good idea in general to visit a dermatologist regularly. I go every month or two. He gives my face a thorough cleaning and checking for about twelve dollars—less expensive than a facial, and a thousand times more effective. He works on broken capillaries with an electric needle, and has a special instrument to force pores to give up oil deposits and other matter. This deep cleaning can't be done by any commercial beauty preparations. Even mine aren't that effective!

The basic rules are simple to remember. Cleanliness first.

Avoid drying or aging the skin. Keep it moist, with moisturizers and creams. Drink as much water as you can; by keeping moisture in your body, you retain moisture in your skin. And keep your skin supple. Leather may be beautiful, but even a calf wouldn't be caught alive with it.

9

Creating an Illusion

Now you've taken care of your skin—but what transforms it? Make-up can be used to disguise or camouflage a multitude of sins. It can correct small eyes, double chins, hanging eyelids, wide noses, and fat faces. It brings a bloom where there was none, shoos small wrinkles out of sight, opens up the eyes. But most women don't understand the corrective uses of make-up at all, what it can do to transform not-so-good features. They still believe it's just a way of applying color to the face.

I'm part of the vanguard of cosmetics producers who believes women should be reeducated. I train my salespeople to do that. And I say to you: Make-up can create an *illusion*. It can take five or ten years off the face. It can change a woman from nondescript to sensational. It's all in knowing how: *Misuse or over-application of make-up can make a woman look older.*

I'd do anything to have the movie star Ann Miller in my hands. I would do her over completely; I would make her so beautiful her head would swim. For she has all the equipment, with flawless skin and large eyes. Her hair is beautiful, but dyed too black now. I'd soften it to dark brown. I'd get rid of her round cheeks by using sculpturing colors. I'd tone down her mouth, soften the accentuation of her eyes. Instead of being camp, she'd be one of the most gorgeous women in the world.

I care how women look, and I try to offer my customers a personal service. Some four hundred of my salespeople are scattered around the country, and I teach them to help a woman plan her individual look, no matter what the trend might be. The salespeople listen because they are paid by The Polly Bergen Company, not by the stores in which they work.

Ten women and two men travel across the United States training all of our people behind the counters. These twelve have been trained by me, and I spend two or three days with them every time I add a new product to the line. I even teach nail care and hair-framing, with products I don't sell (since I don't have a nail or hair line at this time). All this allows my representatives in each store to advise a customer on make-up in relation to the structure of her face, or to teach her little tricks, like minimizing a big nose.

I don't teach women to rely too heavily on make-up. *Many people spend needless hours in applying cosmetics.* There's *no* need for it, and most women don't—or shouldn't—have the time. My make-up routine is normally ten minutes. I can extend it for a more elaborate nighttime look, but for the day, my ten-minute quickie works this way:

- On a clean and dry face, apply moisturizer from hairline down, including neck, throat, and whatever is uncovered by the dress or top you're wearing. I'll say it till I'm hoarse: *Never omit moisturizer!*

- Over the moisturizer apply a very, very thin film of foundation with the hands. Clean fingertips are your best applicator; all others get dirty.

- Blend rouge into cheek. I prefer cream or liquid to powder rouge.

- Lightly dust forehead, eyes, mouth, and chin area with powder, to avoid shininess. (Many women can skip the rouge and powder if they don't need them and save themselves another half minute or so.)

- Now a light touch of eye shadow on each lid and, if you feel like it, a little shadow blended under the lower lashes.

- Mascara usually takes the longest of all to apply well. If you're in a hurry, use an automatic mascara. The final result isn't quite as good, but it will do.

● Lipstick, and you're ready to face the world.

Once you're proficient at this routine, you can do it in seven minutes. Within that time I can add false eyelashes, which I've learned to put on in forty seconds, but it takes a lot of practice. Seven minutes is not much time, and the unannounced guest won't mind waiting.

If he does, or if you're already late for an appointment, or if there's a gang of four-year-olds in the house ready to demand your attention any second, the three-and-a-half-minute routine is for you:

● Apply moisturizer.
● Smooth on eyeshadow and use automatic mascara.
● Apply lipstick.

You may not be your most beautiful or most glamorous, but you *will* have more confidence in yourself. And very young women probably don't need more make-up than this at any time.

The shortcuts are most effective if you've studied your face, if you know exactly what to use on it, where and how to apply. Each part of the face has different problems, different solutions, and needs different cosmetics. All must blend together for a single impression: a more radiant you. But before the entire image is complete, a woman, like a painter, must work on each section individually.

The **foundation** is exactly what its name says: *the first, basic step to creating an illusion.* It should be put on like a second skin, so thinly that it looks as though there's nothing there. If someone says, "Hey, what a terrific foundation you've got on!" then you've failed. They should say, "Hey, what terrific skin you've got!" People say that to me, and I don't have beautiful skin. I don't think I have even good skin. It's very thin, with burst capillaries, splotches, freckles. Under the foundation they're not so noticeable, and the make-up corrects the tone of my skin.

Many women think foundation make-up is a cure-all. It isn't. These women lay on foundation as though they were paving a driveway. Instead of hiding their facial flaws, they're adding ten years to the face. The heavy application settles into every line and wrinkle, emphasizing them. As a matter of fact, the best and easiest way to make a face look much older for character roles in movies and television is to apply a heavy make-up foundation, wrinkle up the face, then powder over.

Foundation is basically formulated to give a skin tone and provide minimum coverage. The proper color is determined by color of hair, eyes, and the natural pigmentation of the skin. Just as there are only four basic colors (brunette, blond, redhead, gray), there are four basic skin tones: peach, yellow, pink, and almost white. The most perfect skin is a balance between beige and peach.

Foundations should be used to correct natural color. They look different on each woman, because every skin reflects its own tint. If, like me, your skin has strong pink or red tones in it, use yellow or beige foundations to balance out the redness toward a peaches-and-cream look. If your skin has too much yellow or whiteness, on the other hand, use pink and peach colors to neutralize the sallowness. Many women have sallow skin, but no one need show it. Very pale or colorless skin should have a pink-red tone for a healthy glow.

The Polly Bergen Company has only a few, basic foundation shades: Fresh Peach, Pure Beige (for reddish skin), Sun Beige (a darker beige for suntans or darker-skinned women), Bronzine (dark beige for deep suntans and black women), Almost White, for the pale evening look, and Pale Ivory, which takes the skin to a porcelain.

Many women can wear a number of these shades. It's important to remember, though most women never think of it at all, that it's not just your *skin pigmentation* but the *color of your clothes* that should determine your foundation. I can, and do, wear all the foundation shades except Almost White and Bronzine, which are too extreme for my coloring. I have a wardrobe of foundation make-ups, and that lets me wear any color I want. No more of that "Gee, it's a great color but I can't wear it, it doesn't go with my complexion."

When I'm wearing red or bright blue I use beige make-up, to tone down the bright colors. When I'm in black, I use pink or peach make-up. Black tends to deaden and drain all color from the face. On sallow skin it's devastation. Yet it doesn't have to be—just add pink or peach. You'll look fine!

White is the opposite: It can be worn by almost everyone, except possibly the woman with very white skin, who must add color first. For a monotone look, I wear a brown or beige dress, beige foundation, chestnutty cheeks, and a brownish lipstick.

I use the foundation to correct skin tone. This means natural pigmentation and reflection of colors from clothes. I use it so no one will *notice* I'm wearing any. I'll let people notice I'm wearing lipstick, and maybe eyeshadow, but that's all. No one should see any correction I've done on my face.

The most important **correction product** in my life is Perfection Stick. It's wonderful for covering brown spots, freckles, and any other less-than-adorable marks on my face. It's applied from the applicator directly to the spots it is to cover. Then, by rolling my finger lightly over the spot, I blend it into the foundation. The other well-known corrective sticks, which I used in show business over the years, are thick as glue, and chalky. They don't move or blend well. They're supposed to cover dark shadows under the eyes, but the concealer is so apparent that it's worse than the shadow.

I use Perfection Stick for *highlighting,* too. It should be one, two, or even three shades lighter than the foundation. Many models work with shading, using dark tones along the sides of the nose and in the cheeks for the sunken-cheek look. This is fine for an expert, but a nonprofessional can wind up looking as though she has five-o'clock shadow.

I prefer to do the reverse: to highlight or spotlight the face, creating lights where the face has become shadowed from expression lines. The philosophy is to accentuate the positive and minimize the negative. I draw attention away from the lines *and* highlight my good points.

There are some secrets in my use of Perfection Stick. It's perfect for a home face lift. The easiest way to lift a face when it begins to droop is by concealing those crevasses around the mouth. When such a wrinkle develops into the Grand Canyon, the skin plumps out around it; light doesn't get into the area, and it creates a shadow on the face. With Perfection Stick, I draw a light line from the corners of the nose to the corners of the mouth, filling in that dark valley with lightness. This gives the illusion of lifting the whole face. It's fantastic, and the rank amateur can do it with astonishing results.

For a wide nose, draw a light line with the stick from the bridge right down the length of the nose. Blend it in. This highlighting draws attention to the bridge of the nose, away from the overall width.

The stick is good for crow's-feet at the corners of the eyes and for the lines between the eyes. It also helps diminish any scars by eliminating the shadow. For laugh lines around the eyes I prefer to use a light make-up instead of the stick, because the area is larger than just crow's-feet or scars.

My next correction is on the neck. I use a base that's a shade or two darker than my foundation and draw a line along my jawbone, because one side of my face has a very indefinite jawbone line, making my profile look fat. I then blend the color down my neck. This throws that area into a darker shadow, creating a more definitive jawline. It's also a good trick for double chins.

One shade difference in make-up, well blended, is so subtle that no one can detect it. But be sure to blend: If make-up stops at the chin, you'll look as if you have a two-tone face and neck.

Next comes **rouge**, which goes *under* the cheekbone. The rouge is darker than my foundation, and it eliminates roundness in my cheeks, giving me a higher-looking cheekbone. The cheekbone itself is very light, and I'll often highlight it with Perfection Stick. This is the reverse of usual beauty advice, which tells you to apply rouge into the cheekbone. I think that's wrong. Rouge should be a corrective in shaping the face, as well as giving youthful color. Properly applied, it sinks in the cheek and gives it a good contour. Of course, women with sunken cheeks should do the reverse: light make-up on the cheek, rouge on the cheekbone.

Never use dry rouge; it makes the cheek look old. Youth is a moist, dewy, shiny cheek. A cheek that's dry and powdered can't be young. Our cream rouge has a faint shimmer in it, to shine on the cheek without being theatrical. We have three shades: Apricot Rosee, Chestnut Spice, and Rich Red. We also have two moisture-blend cheek sticks: Mauve and Nutmeg. All five should blend in easily with the basic foundation colors.

Since my face is wide, I put slightly lighter make-up at the center and darker make-up, including rouge, at the outer edges to throw the border of the face into shadow. This focuses attention on the center, minimizing the width. Narrow or long faces should reverse the procedure.

The last thing I do in preparing the canvas of my face before the dramatic emphasis of eyes and lips is to go over all the areas I've highlighted with a very light **face powder**. This sets the make-up. I use loose powder, not pressed. Pressed powder was invented for touch-ups during the day. It was never formulated to set make-up.

Powder should be totally transparent—no color whatsoever. Color in a powder can undo all the other color that's been put on the face. On top of foundation it can streak or bring the face to an ungodly yellow or orange. Transparent powder goes on any color skin and within a moment takes on the skin tone. It removes the shine and sets the make-up.

If you don't want any powder remaining on your face after the make-up is set, pat a damp sponge lightly all over it. This helps give a moist, dewy look. And *never, never powder your cheeks*. It's the same story as with dry rouge. I powder my eyes for a dry surface. Then I apply **eye shadow**.

Eyes tell their own story. They always do; they're the most expressive feature most of us have. Eyes are magnets. Eyes are doors, pools, and whatever you've got, the eyes have it. Coloring eyes is to make them more outstanding, and to correct their flaws. When you color eyelids, there's a little puffy area just above the crease. About one out of every ten million ladies doesn't have it. The rest of us do, and it's inherited and there's nothing you can do about it, right? Well, not quite. You could have plastic surgery, which is simple and relatively inexpensive. It's also undetectable, because the incision is made directly in the crease. If you can't afford it, are afraid of it, or your eyes haven't yet reached the moment of truth, there are a few simple tricks to minimize the droop, the hooded-cobra look.

The main thing is to apply dark eye shadow into the crease of the eye and on the puffiness itself, then feather it upward. Grays and browns are natural shadow colors. They also help create the impression that the lashes are so thick and luxurious that they're casting a shadow on the lid. A natural shadow would be gray or brown, not electric blue, electric green, lavender, or pink. The darkness pushes in the puffiness by absorbing light instead of reflecting it. I smudge some of the dark shadow just below my lower lash, to give the illusion that my lower lashes are thick and throwing a shadow.

I'll use a lighter color up from the crease, maybe a frosted medium brown. The earth colors give a natural look, as close to my own coloring as possible. At night I can go into greens and blues, because there's a different kind of lighting. And I change my eye make-up according to the darkness or lightness of my skin. So in winter, when I'm pale, I use dark shades around my eyes. The darkness sets my eyes apart from the rest of my pale face. In summer, I do the reverse, making my eyes light against my tanned skin.

I want people to look at my eyes (and *in* my eyes). I decided to make my eyes outstanding, and I think I've succeeded. I can create an illusion. People tell me my eyes are gorgeous. I know they're not, but I've been able to create them.

Until a few years ago I always wore heavy **eyeliner.** But as I got older, I realized it was too hard. At first I looked strange enough without my usual eyeliner for people to ask me if I was ill. That naturally interrupted the experiment immediately. But not permanently; I learned to use shadows in the right way to make a dark frame around my eyes, still emphasizing them, but with a softer, less made-up look.

Women with deep-set eyes should use a very light and frosted eye shadow. The light will pick up the frost and color, pulling the eyes "out." Learning techniques of light and dark can help you correct most common eye problems.

But eye shadow is generally used less as a corrective make-up than as a fashion accessory. The Polly Bergen Company has only a few foundation colors, but many, many eye shadow colors. Eye color need have almost nothing to do with choice of shadow. Many women still believe that shadow color should complement their own; blue-eyed women pick blues and aquas, green-eyed women choose greens, and brown-eyed women go to browns and grays. But women should experiment and change their shadow colors just as they do their clothes and accessories. I have blue eyes and wear brown shadows most of the time, but I also like yellows, greens, pinks, reds, and violets. The more color there is in my skin, the brighter my eye shadow. Generally I try to blend the same tones, but many times I mix them. Flexibility is an important ingredient of beauty.

It's good to remember, though, that too much make-up of any kind will not give the desired effect and might bring about the opposite.

Eyebrows can go darker or lighter. **Eyebrow pencil** is

imperative for the women with no eyebrows. It can also reshape a brow, correcting the contour or thickness. Most brows need clearer definition. Women who bleach their hair should use an eyebrow lightener to give the brows the same color as the hair. Nothing looks worse than a mane of blonde hair above black brows.

To determine length of eyebrow, I use the old pencil trick. I take an ordinary lead pencil and slant it across my face, from nostril up to the outer edge of the eye. Where the pencil extends beyond the eye should be the end of the brow. I learned this trick many years ago from make-up artists at the studios. The brow should begin above the inside corner of the eye. (By "should," I just mean a general guideline.)

Many eyebrows are too low, too close to the eye. Mine were at one time, and it's not beautiful. It closes in the eye, makes it smaller. By **tweezing** the space between eye and brow you open up the eye, making it prettier and larger-looking.

A fashion of the seventies has been the no-eyebrow look. It's a throwback to the thirties and forties. Women pluck their eyebrows almost clean, or even wax them off entirely. But one should remember that, once plucked or waxed, eyebrows won't grow back. Those who were in fashion for the bald eyebrow will be in trouble when thick eyebrows come back.

A woman can experiment with fashion, but individuality comes first. If she looks best to herself with heavy brows and thick lashes, she should certainly stick with them. I think the seventies look of the more naked eye works for me, but I don't for a moment believe it's the answer for everyone. Though my make-up line is available in the newest fashions, I emphasize to my salespeople that a woman's individuality always comes first. They can tell her what's "in," but if the fashion isn't for her, she should stay away from it. I'm not in business to discourage people from new fashions, obviously; but I also don't think it's right to urge people to buy what doesn't suit them.

False lashes go in and out of fashion. As I've said, I never wore them as a young actress, because of a reverse ego. Now I sometimes wear them, sometimes not. At an intimate gathering, a small dinner party, I don't. My own lashes aren't bad, and they aren't outstanding, but they work. And I don't have to dread taking them off in a more intimate situation later.

I'll wear them when I'm going to be photographed, because

strong light really washes out blue eyes. I'll wear them before a large group of people. When I give speeches on tour, I wear them sometimes, and sometimes not. It depends on my mood, how tired I am, and what kind of impact I want to make.

I apply them after **mascara.** First I use cake mascara, which I prefer to the automatic kind because it can be controlled through the amount of dampness on the brush. It should be applied very slowly with an almost dry brush. The dryness prevents lashes caking together. A wet brush, or one with too much mascara on it, glues the lashes together. And whether you're applying false lashes or not, you want the real ones to be separated and still look as thick and full as possible. I use the automatic-mascara dispenser just to touch up my mascara.

The mascara on, I take a little wand or toothpick and apply a tiny film of Duo Surgical Adhesive (Mitchum-Thayer, Inc.) to the base strip of the false lash. Carefully holding the lashes with tweezers, I place them immediately above the natural lashes and press against the edge of the lid. Bottom lashes are more difficult to apply, and less frequently worn. They are applied with adhesive just below the lower lashes and carefully pushed up. Take great care not to injure the eye, eyelid, or lashes, and keep the adhesive well away from the eye itself.

Once the lashes are in place, I take tweezers and squeeze together the false lash and the real one at the base, so they'll entwine. No one can tell where my lash stops and the false one begins.

Mascara is essential for this. False lashes are an artificial color. They're dyed and will never match a real eyelash color. But mascara, which is an artificial color, helps blend the two.

I use lashes that are close to my own in shape, thin but spread on an invisible band so that when I apply them they seem to grow right out of the lid. The individual lashes are all different lengths and spaced at different intervals for a natural effect. When you buy lashes, check them and trim them for both length and width.

My full-scale eye make-up, which I use for special occasions, has seven steps:

● moisturizer
● foundation
● eye shadow

- eyeliner (I sometimes use a light one—pale blue, for instance)
- eyebrow pencil
- mascara
- false eyelashes.

It's not as time-consuming as it sounds. The more you practice, the easier and faster it becomes.

Now my face is almost ready, except for **lipstick.** The one big secret to lipstick is: Always use two colors. A single color is dull, unexciting, and often fades away into nothing, particularly if it's a light frost. If it's a heavy, dark, mat color it contrasts too sharply with skin tones and draws too much attention to the mouth.

The two colors aren't mixed or placed one on top of the other. No, they're coordinated. I like to use five examples for well-coordinated pairs of lipsticks:

red mat and red frost
orange mat and orange frost
nutmeg and pink frost (or orange frost)
pink mat and pink frost
chestnut (deep brown) and fawn frost (sensational for blonds).

To experiment with a new lipstick, first make sure your lips are thoroughly cleaned. Use soap and water or a good cleanser, but make sure the stain of the old lipstick is gone.

Use the darker color first. Spread it on the upper and lower lips. Follow the border of the lip very carefully. If you leave part uncolored, it will be lighter than the rest of the lip and will form a highlight, making the lip appear much fuller or larger. The darker tone tends to make it smaller, just as a white dress makes a woman look heavier and a black dress makes her look more slender.

When the dark color is on nice and thick, remove almost all of it from the center of the lips with a tissue, leaving only the dark border around the edge of the lips. Now apply the lighter color or frost to the central part of the lips, blending with the darker color but not bringing it right to the lipline.

You'll have softer, more petulant lips. The highlight in the center brightens the entire mouth.

The final touch is **lip gloss.** This is more than a shine; it's also a treatment to soften the lips. The moisturizer in it keeps lips from chapping and drying out. It even penetrates lipstick.

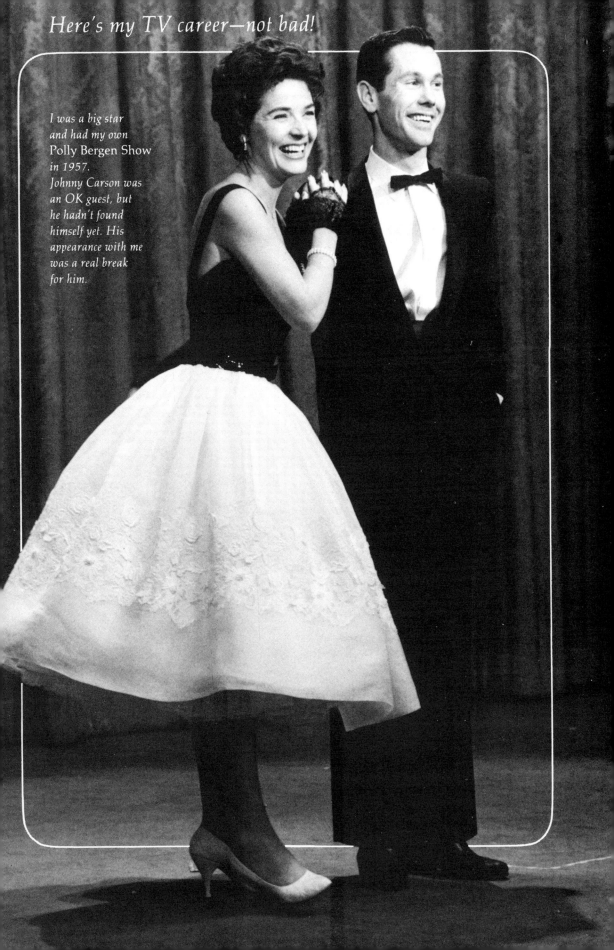

Here's my TV career—not bad!

I was a big star
and had my own
Polly Bergen Show
in 1957.
Johnny Carson was
an OK guest, but
he hadn't found
himself yet. His
appearance with me
was a real break
for him.

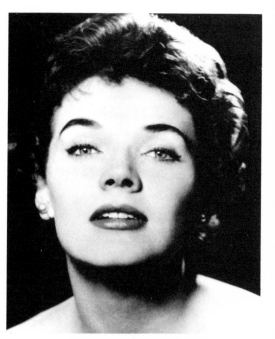
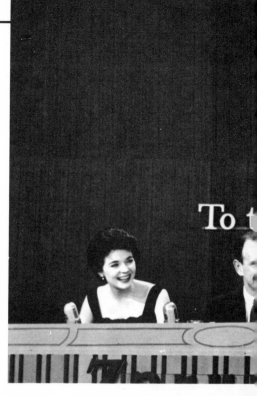

To t

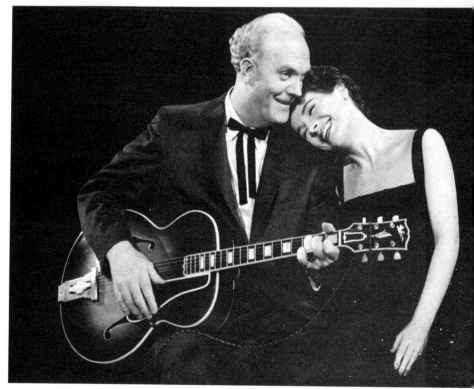

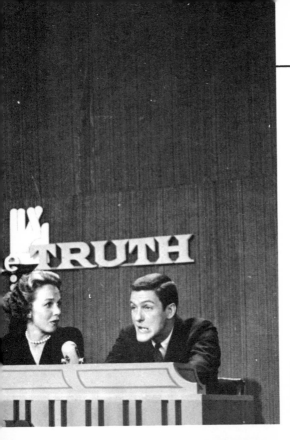

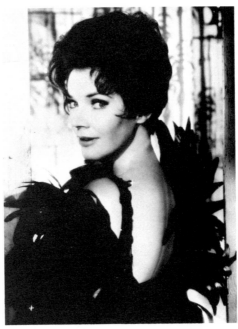

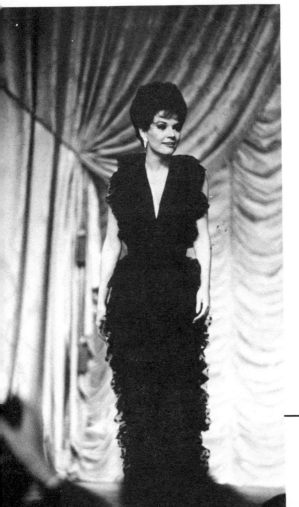

Now I'm really moving. Ava Gardner had been another of my early idols (opposite, top left), but I finally started growing up when I became a top night-club singer (above) and started doing fashion shows (left). When I had Daddy performing on my own show, I just about flipped (opposite page). But I suppose that nothing built me up more as a celebrity than five years as a resident character on To Tell the Truth.

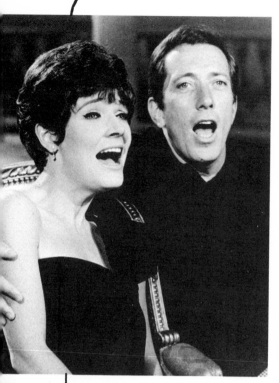

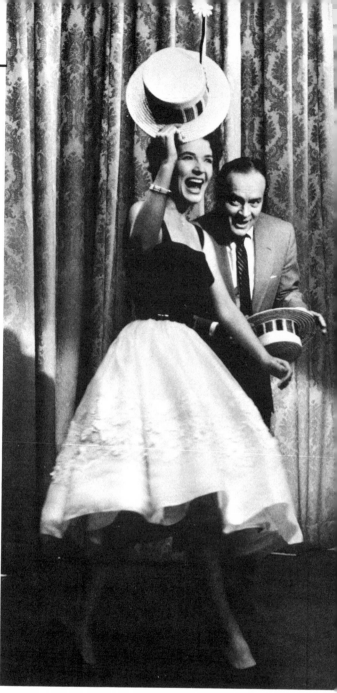

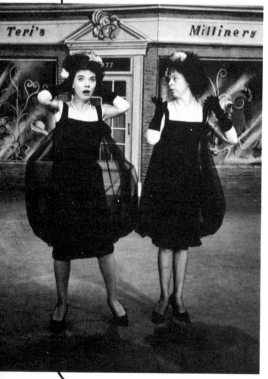

Going strong on TV with Andy Williams, Bob Hope, and Carol Hainey (this page) and keeping up (opposite) with Joey Bishop, Red Skelton, and—heaven help us!—Richard Chamberlain on Dr. Kildare. You can see that I was no longer exactly shy. I certainly knew how to pour it on at stage center for occasions like the grand finale on one of my own TV specials (bottom, extreme right).

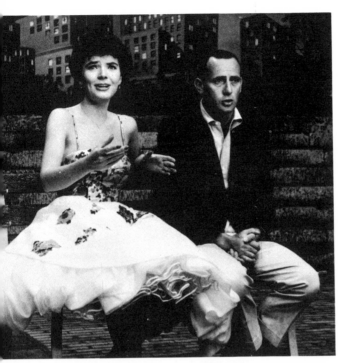

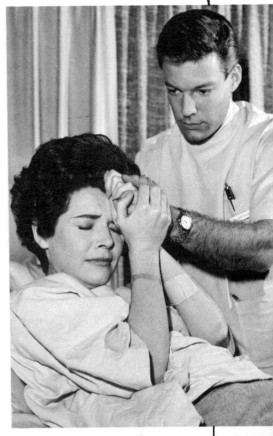

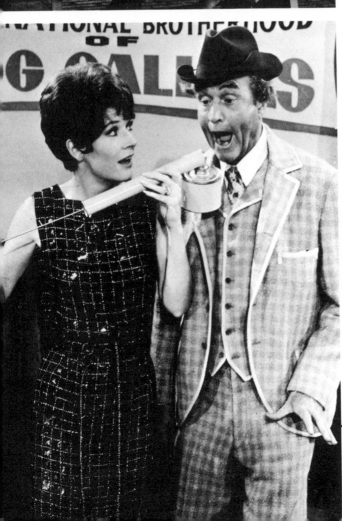

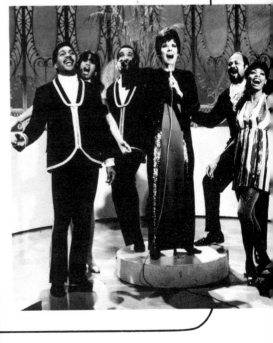

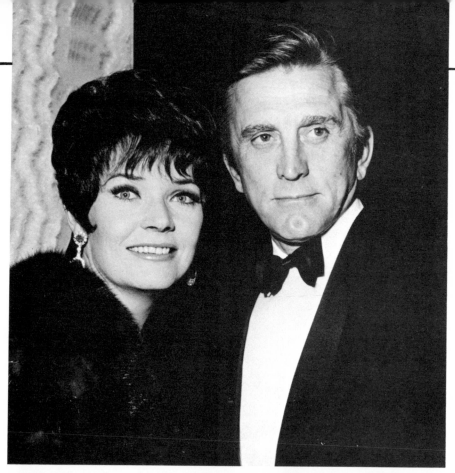

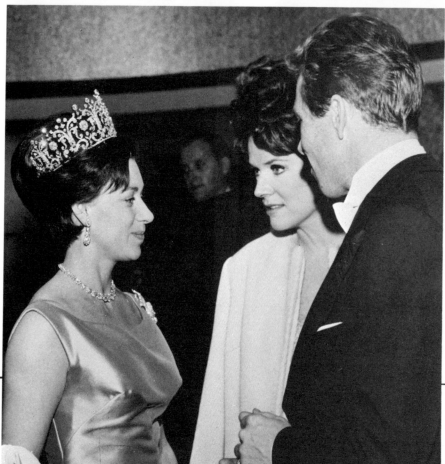

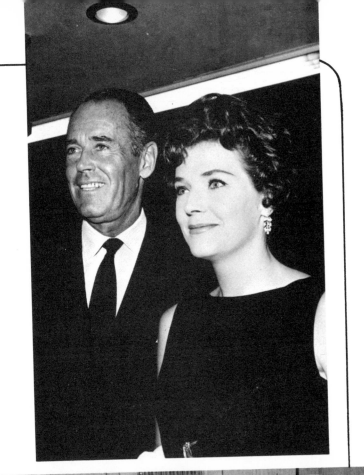

My social life didn't exactly make me Miss Wallflower, either. On the opposite page I'm at a premiere with Kirk Douglas and chatting with Princess Margaret and Lord Snowdon at a benefit I chaired. I was seen with Henry Fonda (right) and took my place in the Beverly Hills housewives' and hostesses' "Mafia," which included such friends as (bottom, left to right) Barbara Rush, Mrs. Kirk Douglas, and Janet Leigh.

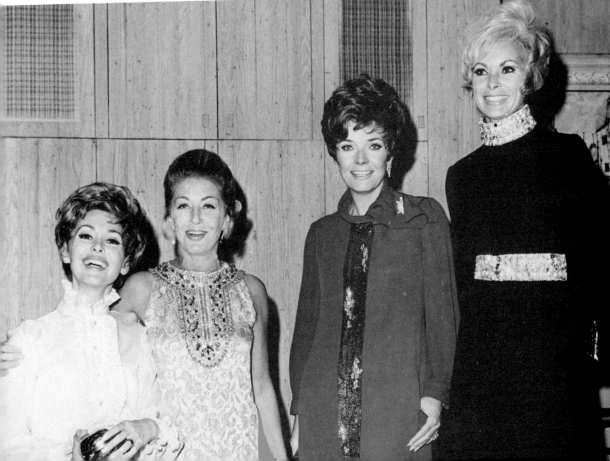

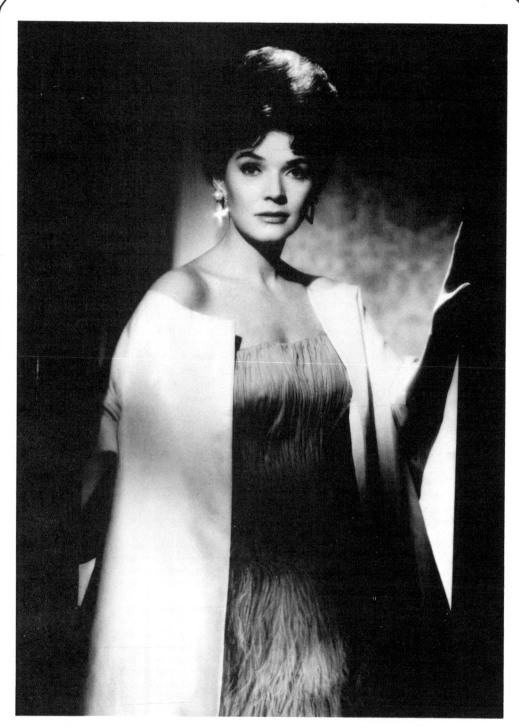

Even as a big-time star, I couldn't resist the temptation to overdress.

Use a lip gloss even if you're not wearing lipstick, to keep your lips moist and appealing. On lipstick it adds a sexy look.

Lipstick was once opaque; now it's transparent enough for the lips to be seen through it. The mouth is back. The very pale graveyard look is gone and colors are brighter, prettier than they were. The beiges have become more pink, and earth tones are also popular. Indelible lipstick belongs back in the dark ages when it was shocking for lipstick to be seen on a man's face. We're that much freer now, and people don't care about lipstick one way or the other.

Experiment with colors. There are no fixed rules except that the darker color *always* goes first. Use lipsticks, lip crayons, or pencils. Use a lipstick brush to enlarge the size of your mouth—or to make it smaller—and learn to wield it with the dexterity of Norman Rockwell. The darker mat color should be applied a fraction beyond the lipline. Don't follow the cupid's bow of the upper lip. Gradually, slowly eliminate that little cleft altogether. This will give the mouth fullness.

To extend the lower lip, blend lipstick into the surrounding skin as skillfully as possible, erasing the definite border. The middle of the lip should be heavily made up, then blended out gradually.

Try all sorts of different colors. Don't stick with old styles just because they once were effective. Don't follow the fashion if it doesn't suit you. Change your make-up to coordinate with your wardrobe and—*very important*—learn to change your make-up when you change the color of your hair.

I've changed Ann-Margret's style of make-up and hairdo four separate times. When she had dark auburn hair, I had to tone down the orange in her make-up; it was too harsh with the red overtones in her hair. I kept her skin slightly darker than normal (she was tanned) with a beige-rose tone. Then I surrounded her eyes with brown and green to give her a natural-redhead look. Her mouth I made chestnutty, almost the same color as her hair. The lashes were very dark brown, almost an off-black but not too hard.

I saw her some time later at a party—but she was reddish blond! She greeted me cheerfully: "Hi, Polly. I love your make-up. How does it work with my new hair?"

"Terrible," I told her.

"Why?"

"Well look, I gave you that make-up when your hair was dark. It doesn't work for you as a blond."

Next day she came to my house, and we spent two hours redoing her make-up. I brought her skin tone up much lighter, despite her tan, into a fresh peach color. The former pink tones were too strong against the hair, now blond. I made her eyes look more blue by replacing the tawny brown-greens with grays and blues. I lightened the eyelashes for a softer effect and gave her a peachy-pink lipstick.

It's all common sense. When a woman changes the color of her hair, she must check her make-up. If you repaint your living room, you make sure the new color doesn't look horrible with the old fabric of the furniture or the draperies.

A last word on make-up: It doesn't have to be limited to the face and neck. A mole or wart can be made into a beauty mark with an eyebrow pencil. Body paint can be fun, amusing. It depends on the place and the person. I never got much into rouging knees, but that's because I'd like to overlook my legs altogether. Rouging the nipples can be a turn-on for some men, and for some women. It can turn you on yourself. It either works or it doesn't. It's silly, I know, but fun to try once in a while.

The old show-business stunt of rouging the cleavage will give the impression of your breasts being much larger. The rouge is darker than your own skin, so it increases the shadow effect between the breasts and makes the valley appear deeper. I used to do it all the time when I was in show business, wearing evening gowns on stage. That gave my breasts a fuller, more *saftig* look. That *saftig* look was very important in those days, and people came up to me saying, "I've been a fan of yours all my life, Polly Bergman," or: "Polly Berger, I've loved you since I was a little kid."

I don't use that trick any more. I'm not as concerned about being put-together as I once was. Make-up is fine, and it makes you look prettier, but it can also make you look older. At least to the point of no return, in your fifties or sixties, when the natural look won't do much for you. But I still have a few good years, and I can go without any make-up at all. Until a year ago I would've sworn I wasn't as attractive to men without make-up. But last summer, on the raft trip down the Colorado River with Peter and P.K., I didn't wear a speck of make-up. My eyes are half their size without make-up, but I had a clean-scrubbed look that made me seem much younger. I met a man on the trip, almost ten years younger than I. The way he looked at me convinced me my naked face could be just as appealing, for I realized I looked softer, more vulnerable than when made up.

That's a kind of beauty, unsophisticated, very free. It's not for all women, and not for all occasions. But nothing in the world would fit that bill. Each of us must discover how to look as good as *she* can possibly look, and adapt that for the occasion, the man and, most of all, herself. To that one woman in a million who always looks breathtakingly sensational in no make-up at all, I say: God bless you.

10

Give Yourself a Hand

At twenty-seven, I was in films but I had no fingernails. Whenever I was nervous—which was most of the time—I gnawed my fingernails. I couldn't stand to look at them. They were repulsive to me, and I figured they must be twice as awful to other people. I clasped my hands together a lot, not in prayer, but to hide my nails.

They were a real mess until I met Nena Rico, a brilliant manicurist who owns the Nails by Nena manicure salons in New York and Beverly Hills. Her specialty, aside from giving the best manicures I've ever seen, is educating women in nail care. I like to think I graduated from her course *magna cum laude.*

I'm proud of my nails now, unbelievably proud. I can look at my hands often. I like to; but even if I didn't want to, I couldn't miss my hands—and neither can any woman. A woman's hands are the most visible part of her except for her face. In almost every activity of life her hands are on view, to herself and to others.

In a sense they are calling cards. Hands give out a lot of messages about your personality immediately. The first contact (after the visual one) that people have with each other is usually shaking hands. A paw with chipped, uncared-for nails is a turn-off. Chewed nails are a giveaway for the insecure, uptight lady. Hangnails and frazzled cuticles are real downers. Flaky nail polish, white spots, and uneven nails undermine the well-groomed appearance. But there's no need to let this happen, because with only a little time and effort any woman can transform an ugly hand into a great asset. There's no excuse why every woman can't enjoy seeing beautiful hands every time she looks at her own.

The first thing to remember about having beautiful nails is to keep all ten of them at equal lengths. That length will vary with individuals, though as a general rule you should keep the part that extends beyond the finger no more than *one-third* the length of the entire fingernail. If your fingernail from cuticle to quick is half an inch long, the additional nail should be one quarter inch. You don't have to get out a ruler—it's just a general guideline.

Now consider the *type and shape* of your nails. Are they dry and brittle? Do the ends split and break easily? Then they're like mine, and like millions of women's. What's their shape? Wide, narrow? Long, short? Rounded or flat, turned up or turned down? Are they round-tipped or square-tipped, are they oval or round? No matter—each can be beautiful, though each must be treated differently.

Even extremely narrow or tubular nails can be clipped, filed, and enameled to give them individuality. The smart woman takes advantage of the distinctiveness of her own nails and heightens it. Though each woman has her own specific problems and ways of dealing with her nails, here are some commonsensical do's and don't's which will help most women in achieving beautiful nails:

Ten Do's

- Try to have a manicure once a week. If not at a salon, train yourself to do your own expert manicuring.

- Wear gloves when doing the dishes or other housework that might injure or break your nails.

- Learn to dial the telephone with your knuckles, or use a plastic dialer or the eraser end of a lead pencil.

- After a manicure, keep your fingers out of water for as many hours as possible to harden the enamel. Twelve hours is ideal, though most women will not be able to do this.

- Learn to pick up coins and other small objects by sliding them along the surface of a table to the edge and then grasping them without using the nail.

- If you break nails when putting on girdles or pantyhose, wear plastic or cotton gloves. They protect the nails and prevent tearing or puncturing of undergarments.

- Use a good nail cream as often as possible when you retire at night.

- Push back cuticles with a soft face cloth when taking a bath, or with a bath towel when drying off.

- Use nail clippers for trimming fingernails—never scissors.

- Learn to patch your own nails.

Ten Don't's

- Don't smoke. In addition to everything else smoking does, it dries out and discolors nails.

- Never open jewelry clips and clothes snaps with your fingernails.

- Never *ever* bite your nails.

- Don't suck your nails, either—that nervous habit is as destructive as biting.

- Never use a sharp instrument to clean under the nail.

- Avoid all metal nail-treatment instruments (except for clippers).

- Don't let polish remain on the nails for more than ten days.

- Never cut the cuticle for any reason whatsoever.

- Remove all old polish before putting on any more.

- Don't file the sides of the nails—that weakens them.

Not every woman can afford the time or cost of a regular manicure appointment. *But she* can *teach herself the basic steps of a professional manicure.* After studying what Nena has done to my nails over a year, I can give myself a better manicure than those available in most beauty shops.

As I said, my nails are flaky and brittle. I also get white spots on them, from small bruises through contact with hard objects.

Automobile door handles have broken off every one of my nails several times. I've even written to car manufacturers in Detroit, begging them to invent a handle that isn't designed to ruin the nails of every woman in the country. So far they haven't been very receptive. And it's curious that the more expensive a car—especially foreign models like Rolls-Royce and Mercedes—the worse the door handles. That doesn't mean you have to refuse the Silver Cloud on Christmas morning because of your nails, but mind the handles when you step into the next custom-made one.

In the meantime, have someone else open the car door whenever possible. Or leave the window open and reach in to the easier-operating handle inside. (Of course, you might find some things missing from your car if you do this, but your hands will stay lovelier!)

Educating hands isn't easy, but it can be done. I've taught myself to use the balls of my fingers for almost all activities, especially picking things up. Constant vigilance is the price to pay for good hands, and eventually that vigilance will become second nature. Start by turning light switches off and on with the knuckles or heel of the hand instead of fingertips. I've even learned to fasten jewelry with the balls of my fingers.

Once a woman accustoms herself to not using her nails for anything utilitarian—not even to scratch mosquito bites—she should keep her nails clean. They are the biggest germ collectors we have, even worse than hair. Keep a nail brush by your bath, another at the kitchen sink.

When I wear gloves, the plastic or rubber kind, I rub a little nail and cuticle cream on first. The combination of heat and moisture works wonderfully.

Every week or ten days I give myself a manicure, trying to set one night apart for it. You don't need a *whole* evening for nails, of course, but it's easier to get the job done if you've specifically taken the time for it.

The first thing I do is set up a tray beside a comfortable chair in my bedroom, right smack in front of the television set. Then I fill the tray with cotton balls, an orange stick or two, several emery boards, polish remover, Q-tips, cuticle cutters, metal nail clippers, padded nail buffer, paper and cotton patches, and a pumice stick. From the refrigerator I bring enamel, base coat, and ceramic finish coat. (I always keep nail polish in the refrigerator; it keeps the enamel thin and easy to apply.)

The tray's set up. I leave it and have a leisurely bath—with bath oil, of course, and maybe bubbles too. While in the tub I push back the cuticles firmly but gently. Once I'm dried off and moisturized—and there's a great old movie going on the TV set—I plop down in the chair and get to work on my hands, which are thoroughly dry.

Step 1. Preparing the nails: Dip a Q-tip in polish remover. Bring it as far underneath the nail as possible to remove all coats of sealer, enamel, and/or polish from the previous manicure. Then use an orange stick with a small amount of cotton on the tip; dip it into the remover and work carefully under the nail. Once the underside of the nail is satisfactorily clean, use cotton balls immersed in polish remover for the main part. Cotton is twice as effective as tissues.

Step 2. Cleaning the nails: With the polish off, I can see the true condition of each nail and cuticle. With cuticle cutters, I carefully trim off any hangnails, making sure I never cut the cuticle at all. I check each nail for white spots and ridges. The ridges can be minimized with the buffer stroked horizontally against the grain of the nails and always in one direction. But I'm careful not to buff too hard or too long. Heat from the friction is damaging and drying to the nail. Next I soak my nails in lotion—if it's slightly heated, so much the better. You can use many creams and lotions for this; even a cream moisturizer is good. And one of the very best soakers of all is warm olive oil—great for the nails. Dry off nails and gently push back the cuticle with a soft cloth. For the woman fortunate enough not to have to wear enamel (which necessarily means she won't use patches), the manicure is almost over. She'll file her nails, then perhaps use a glaze or colorless polish. But I go on to my next step.

Step 3. Patching: I call this *nail saving.* I've had the entire end of a fingernail break off and fall to the floor and I've picked it up, saved it for my manicure, and then patched it back on the growing nail. I make the covering patches from paper used to filter coffee. It's thin and enormously strong. I cut a suitable patch to start below the torn or weak part of the nail and often carry it right over the tip, folding and trimming it.

When I need even stronger support for a broken nail, I use a cotton patch. Taking a fluff of cotton from a ball, I flatten it out and twist the ends a little so it won't come apart. Then I trim it to size, conforming to the contour of the nail. Both type patches can be glued on with special nail cement which can be bought at almost any nail counter.

I prepare the patches ahead of time, and like to have a supply of both kinds on hand. If you don't have the time or energy to make your own patches, you can always buy them.

Once the patch is on and dried, I often use the pumice-stone stick on the rough skin at the sides of my nails, to get rid of calluses and dry areas where the skin is building up or flaking off.

Step 4. Filing: Use only an emery board to file nails, never a metal file. First I'll use metal clippers (*not* scissors) to get my nails the length I want. The clippers only cut; they're much too awkward to be used for shaping.

As Nena Rico taught me, I *never* file the sides of the nails. I shape the tip gently with the fine-grain side of the emery board, *always* filing in one direction: away from the cuticle and toward the tip. Going back against the grain leaves tiny weak spots where cracking and peeling will begin. When I'm through filing, I test with the balls of my fingers for any sign of jaggedness. I continue to use the emery board until every infinitesimal rough spot is gone.

After all filing is over, wipe nails off with a slightly damp cloth or tissue to remove the fine dust. This is particularly important if polish is used, because in the filing process by emery board, minute particles could clog under polish and give a lumpy or grainy look.

Step 5. The base coat: Use a good brand of clear polish. The best have an oil base to prevent dryness. Do the underneath part of the nail first, making sure the polish comes right up and over the edge of the nail. Then cover the top of the nail in long, even strokes. Repeat with a second coat. For each coat on the top of the nail, there should be a coat underneath. The nail tip should be covered because, as the striking edge, it is the first part of the nail to chip and break.

Step 6. Color coat: I begin underneath the nail tip so the enamel oozes out over the tip. When I put the top layer on, it smoothes the tip, leaving a coat on the very edge. By the time I've finished the first coat on all nails, the first hand is dry enough for me to start on the second. The longer you allow each coat to dry, the better. It's just the time to catch up on television.

After the second color coat is on, contemplate the shape of your nails. I always avoid a pointed tip. Everyone should; it's too clawlike. It's most harmonious and balanced if the tip matches the shape at the cuticle. But sometimes that won't work, I know.

Step 7. Sealer: It isn't enough to protect the nail with enamel; the *enamel itself* must be protected from chipping. Use a sealer. I like Ceramic Glaze best; it's hard and gives final protection and strength.

Step 8. Final buffing: Use a buffer on the sealing coat only after it's dried thoroughly. Buffing gives an extra finishing touch that makes nails glow.

It's over! I have a total of *ten* coats of polish, five over and five under each nail: two coats of base polish, two coats of color, and the final sealer coat, all going above and below the nails. They provide super protection, to withstand daily knocks and pressure.

The manicure *does* take some time. It all gets down to whether you want beautiful nails or not. There's always some price to pay for beauty—in this case, time and a little extra patience. No matter what sort of nails a woman has, they can be beautiful if she follows my instructions.

I'll go without make-up to rest my face, but I'd never leave my nails unenameled. The last time I tried, I lost three nails. Those ten coats of polish are like a suit of armor, and my nails need it in their everyday battles.

Each woman has her own color preference. Some choose a natural, light pink shade. Others go in for the kooky, far-out greens, blacks, yellows, blues, while some add decals. Many women match their nails to their lipstick, which isn't a bad idea. I like deep shades of red and pink or burgundy for winter and fall, when my clothes are darker, and lighter shades in spring and summer. I choose a color that will go with as many of my clothes and color preferences as possible. If a woman has time to change the color of her nails with each outfit, good luck to her. That's a real beauty trap. I certainly don't have that kind of time, and I doubt that other women have either.

But beware of time-savers, too. The worst of all are certain fake nails made of a substance similar to that used in dental work for temporary fillings. It's a powder-and-liquid mix that extends over a woman's real fingernail on a piece of aluminumlike paper. When it dries it becomes cement and can be filed to the desired shape. (These are not the same as plastic nails, which are glued on for short periods.) I have friends who lost every nail on their hands. These fake nails inhibit the growth of natural nails and should be avoided altogether.

There is no ten-minute nail-care treatment. You'll need one hour for your manicure. But every woman can grow her own healthy nails, *if* she will give them the proper care. If you think you deserve a beautiful hand, give yourself one.

And, while you're at it . . .

ADD A FOOT OR TWO

I do my toenails every three or four weeks, and a pedicure doesn't take any more than twenty minutes. I push the cuticle back, in the bath or afterward. I clip the nails with a toenail clipper, not too short, just slightly below the tip of the toe. I then use an emery board on them so there are no rough edges, but I keep them fairly square. That's the healthiest shape; ingrown toenails result from cutting away the sides.

I separate my toes with a foam-rubber separator, or I use a couple of tissues twisted between each toe. I then apply two coats of base coat and two of color.

When I can, I try to get in to a chiropodist. For a time I wore no polish on my toes, and then I had to go to him more often. My nails, particularly on the big toe, build up and get ridgy. Chiropodists work with something like a sanding machine to remove layers of nail. The sanding also gets rid of white spots, which I have. I think I get them from hitting my toes because I go barefoot all the time. The first thing I do when I get into the house is remove my shoes. My barefoot Southern upbringing!

Luckily, my feet are very healthy. I have no calluses or corns. I'm on my feet all the time and I adore walking. I will not wear shoes that hurt my feet, I *simply* will not. And I believe any woman who does is insane.

Comfort may not be beauty, but where there's discomfort, beauty can't exist. A lovely woman is one who is relaxed and comfortable with herself. She knows both the price and the value of beauty. She may take a whole hour to do her nails, but she won't allow her feet to hurt for one second. We all make compromises and choose priorities. In beauty, the compromises are with fashion, and the priorities go to those things that will make us feel more beautiful, more secure, so that we can forget about ourselves, knowing we look as good as we can, and go on with the business —and joy—of living to the full.

11

Crowning It

Just as make-up must suit hair, so hair must suit your facial structure and life style. The most gorgeous hairdo isn't worth a cent if a woman can't manage it herself. Any woman who goes to the hairdresser every other day should be shot. The hairdresser should be shot. He and she together are creating a dependency that's destroying the woman's life. In this time of wash-and-wear hair, every woman should learn to do her own. She must find a style that not only suits her, but that she can handle. Dependence on other people is torture.

I'm one of the few women in my business who travels all over the world without a hairdresser. I can't cut my hair myself, so when it becomes too uneven I have it cut. When I'm home and have the time, I have my hair done once a week. Otherwise I have it done when I can, which might be once a month.

Over the years I've learned what's best for my hair. A hairdresser who has never seen me before in his life can't possibly know more about my hair than I do. If I walk into a shop and the hairdresser pays no attention to what I say, I walk out again. He's like an interior decorator who completely ignores the taste of the person with whom he's working. I've lived with my hair for forty-three years and know a lot more about it than some idiot who's seeing it for the first time.

I have two hairdressers, one in New York and one in Beverly Hills. I like and trust both of them, because they trust me. They don't fight my natural instincts about my hair. In Beverly Hills it's Guy Richards, one of the most marvelous hairdressers in the country and one of my closest friends. In New York it's Pierre Hambur, also great and very versatile—except that he's recently moved to Phoenix, Arizona. I've learned a lot about hair in general, and my hair in particular, from both men. That's partly because they haven't fought me.

Women can and should learn from hairdressers. Don't bury yourself in a magazine while your hair is being done. Watch and study. Insist on hairdos you can manage, particularly if you're a working woman. Discuss your life style with the hairdresser. How much time do you have for your hair every day? Every week? What's entailed in keeping the hairdo you've chosen? How long can you go without returning to the salon? What would you do if your hairdresser disappeared/died/changed professions?

I keep my hair short, because that's the way it looks best on me and is easiest to manage. I can brush it forward, backward, wear bangs or not. But the basic shape remains the same. If I had one beauty wish it would be to have my hair long, to wear it high in a chignon. That's the chicest look I know, but it doesn't suit me. Some women can wear their hair long or short, going from one to the other and looking great in both. Candy Bergen and Ann-Margret are two perfect examples. The rest of us aren't so lucky.

As a general rule, long hair on women over forty looks awful, unless it's worn in an upsweep or chignon. Otherwise, hanging hair coupled with hanging skin emphasizes downward lines and draws attention to sag and lines. The long, flowing, outdoor look was intended for sixteen-year-olds at the beach. Long hair always offers more variety than short, but short hair is *easier* to maintain. My hair dries in twenty to twenty-five minutes. Very long hair can take an hour and a half, with luck. I can color, wash, and set my own hair in two hours.

The style of hair must fit the woman's *own* personal style. If she comes to her hairdresser with a photograph from a magazine, saying, "I want to look like that," she's probably fooling herself. And the hairdresser should discourage her. Perhaps he can modify the style to suit her, but chances are the shape of her face is different from the model's.

I learned my lesson during the last difficult year of my marriage to Freddie. I was dating men younger than myself, and I wanted to look less sophisticated, more free. I wanted an undone appearance, without hair spray, without backcombing.

I went to Guy and asked him to cut my hair very short, then to give what was left a body permanent, even though I have naturally curly hair. He looked at me peculiarly. I insisted, explaining that I wanted not to have to do anything with my hair. I got my permanent. My head was covered with tiny screw curls, a straight Afro. Hideous. Somehow I managed to exist that way for a full eighteen hours. Then I had my hair straightened.

I asked Guy how he could have allowed me to do a thing like that. "I knew you needed the change emotionally," he said, "and nothing I could have said would've stopped you."

He was absolutely right. Now my hair is loose, short, and airy. It's very soft when it's clean, but after two days—with a little dirt—it has great body and falls into the right waves. It lasts from one setting to the next, and I rarely cover it with a hat.

I use a minimum of spray, just sufficient to hold the height of my hair. Every night I brush it out completely. Hair without spray feels much better and is more sensual than a lacquered mass. If you spray your hair into a solid form, it means Hands Off! and no man will want to touch it. It's part of the closeup test: Heavily lacquered hair may look marvelous in long shot, but up close it's a turn-off.

In general, whatever makes the hair look more natural is the best choice. But that doesn't mean you should go without color. I've been using color since I was sixteen—I don't remember what it was, but probably an old-fashioned henna red. I was quite gray at eighteen. My father's hair was white when he was twenty, and my mother's hair was salt and pepper at an early age. I inherited the trait, and today my hair would be completely gray if I didn't color it.

When I entered the movies I had henna coloring. At Paramount they made my hair blond-red, because the studio had an excess of Rita Hayworth–type falls and wigs and wanted to use them. In New York I earned the epithet "apricot-thatched." Back in Hollywood, at MGM, I was made a dark brownette when Eleanor Parker decided she wanted to be the only redhead in *Fort Bravo.*

The darker hair turned out to be better for me than the light red. With my pale skin, I'd have had to use too much make-up to give myself color so my face wouldn't look washed out. The dark hair contrasted with my skin and blue eyes, and I could wear less make-up.

Now I use a medium ash-brown rinse without any hint of red. There's so much red in my skin now from being out in the sun that reddish hair would be ridiculous. I color my own hair, using a rinse rather than a dye or bleach. Either of those would leave a red cast to my hair. When I put on the rinse, I isolate wisps of hair so they remain highlighted. No natural head of hair is a single shade; there are always gradations of tone and shading. A solid color gives the hair a hard, unnatural look.

I leave the rinse on for anywhere from ten to twenty-five minutes, depending on how dark I want to go. (And that often depends on my skin color.) For the hair at the back of my head, I lean forward and feel around, parting my hair with my hands. I use a plastic tube applicator, covering the hair as I go. Then I wrap up the hair in a plastic baggie.

Rinse is a temporary color, and disappears gradually with each washing. How long it lasts depends on how well an individual's hair retains color. By the fifth or sixth washing, my hair has lost the color completely, though the darker I've taken the rinse, the longer it lasts.

Since rinses will come out, they're the best form of color to experiment with. Try highlighting brown hair with a soft, streaking effect to give more variation. If you have olive skin with dark eyes, shining brown hair should look beautiful on you. If you have dark hair and sallow skin, keep the hair color and change the skin tone through foundation.

Blonds with yellowish skin tones look good with darker hair color and beige make-up. If you have very fair skin, light lashes and brows, pale eyes, and mousey-colored hair, try a red or light russet rinse. Or simply a soft medium brown.

If your natural hair color doesn't blend with your eyes, skin, and eyebrows, try changing it a little. It's usually a good idea to stay close to the original tone; just make it more interesting. Don't be afraid of a rinse; it's almost like a vegetable coloring, and will always come out.

Dye is indelible. Both dye and bleach are permanent; they grow out only when the hair grows out, leaving the roots. Dyes (tints) darken the hair. They involve only one process and are used mainly on brown and red hair, to deepen the color or cover up gray. Everyone's hair fades as they get older, through natural oxidation and bleaching by the sun. Dyeing the hair restores the color. But never dye your hair black! It's too harsh on everyone; go into a very dark brown instead.

Bleaching is a two-step process. First the hair must be stripped (bleached) and then a toner (color) is added. Gray hair can easily be made blond. Every woman can be the sort of blond she wants to be, but it will look best if her skin tones are light or golden. The olive- or dark-skinned woman should limit herself to blond highlights. Blond hair requires more attention than darker colors. The new hair coming up the shaft is dark, and roots will be visible very quickly. Don't go from dark brown to platinum unless you expect (and can afford) to have your color done every week. (Though I must admit I've seen some natural brunettes who look sensational as blonds, particularly with deep golden tans. But they worked on it.)

Tans on redheads look incongruous, and are a giveaway. Natural redheads usually freckle. If they tan at all, it's not the deep, even tan of a brunette or sometimes a blond. Sometimes very fair-skinned women can look outstanding as brunettes.

The best hair color contains different shades. Not zebra stripes, but soft gradations and highlights. The blatant platinum is out; soft, mixed shades of blond, from almost white to light brown, gives the most soft and natural appearance. Redheads have a wide range of shades too, but they should remember as they grow older not to have the hair quite as red as it was when they were young.

Brunettes can have a field day with tones and highlights, lighter and darker shades, red and blond tones. Gray hair can be darkened or lightened—*not* turned blue or violet—and still have highlights.

Hair that's been colored is dryer than natural hair, so it needs extra **conditioning.** A conditioner should be put on the ends of your hair while the roots are being colored. Oil conditioners are very good. Put it on before you shampoo, leave it a while, then wash out. Or give yourself a hot oil treatment, using a plastic bag or plastic wrap around the head to retain body heat.

You don't need fancy or expensive products. Olive oil is fabulous for dry hair, and whole-egg mayonnaise is my favorite tonic. I keep the mayonnaise on my head for as long as possible before shampooing (overnight would be best, but you have to be alone). It takes a lot of shampooing to get the stuff out, but it's worth it. The hair feels soft and silky. Then set your hair with beer; it gives body. Don't worry about the odor; for some reason, the beer smell completely disappears when the hair dries.

Permanents and straighteners are as drying for the hair as color. If you need to have a permanent or straightening, have it *before* you color. Otherwise, the chemicals from the solution will discolor your hair.

Permanents are not what they used to be, and most women have them to give more body to the hair, more volume. A body permanent uses the largest rods possible, making a loose wave. With straightening, no rods at all are used; the chemical solution is put on and the hair is combed straight.

Though you can color, straighten, set, condition your hair at home, *and* give yourself a permanent, *never* try to cut your own hair. It's guaranteed disaster. You can't get the levels and layers that a hairdresser can, you won't be able to check for evenness, and the back of your head may look as though you stepped into a paper-shredding machine. That's one experiment to stay away from. Always.

And if, after all your care, your hair's *still* a mess, wear a wig. Or wear one when you don't have time to fix your hair, when you're traveling, when you're suddenly called by your office or your child's school, when your husband invites you for lunch in fifteen minutes. But don't wear wigs all the time. Hair must breathe to be healthy. In selecting a wig, choose one that matches your own hair. You can get good wigs now for as little as five dollars. The new fibers can be cut, cleaned with Woolite, dried in twenty minutes, thrown into a plastic bag, and never lose their shape.

Wigs can enhance illusion or be part of corrective disguise. It depends very much on your approach to them. You can have a wig for emergencies but don't always rely on it. You can wear one for fun, even going into a totally different color than your usual one. If you want to be a redhead for one night, or a dazzling blond, it's far better to wear a wig than to subject your hair to harsh chemicals. If you're bald, you wear a wig out of necessity.

But it's best if your crowning glory *is* your own. Beauty means working with what you have, minimizing the bad, emphasizing the good. A wig isn't drastic, of course, but if it's used as disguise, it comes close to the possible pitfalls of plastic surgery.

12

Scalpel, Anyone?

The most radical beauty treatment of all is plastic surgery. It can undo the mistakes that God hath wrought, like flat chests, bulbous noses, or receding chins, or it can work against the ravages of time as it lifts and peels. I've said throughout this book that a woman should accept herself, work with what she's got, and that seems to throw out the possibility of plastic surgery. But it doesn't *have* to, so long as a woman is not deceiving herself.

If she thinks that at forty she can be twenty, forget it. If she thinks she can undergo surgery without having to pay for it in some way, besides money, she should forget that too. Plastic surgery is basically an exchange system. You take a scar instead of a wrinkle. You have your breast reduced, but you still can't go topless. You have your face peeled, but there's a line of demarcation at the throat. Everything has a price, and you must be emotionally ready to trade.

If you are, go ahead. Try. If what's bothering you can be made acceptable through surgery, do it. You don't have to accept a bulbous or hooked nose. You don't have to go through the physical and psychological discomfort of a fifty-inch bustline. If you're not hung up with your wrinkles or your breasts or your nose, hurrah. But if you are, and if you feel so self-conscious about your appearance that it's changing your personality, plastic surgery is legitimate.

If something is standing between you and happiness, change

it. A woman looks in the mirror and all she sees is a nose she can't abide. It doesn't seem to bother anyone else (they may be seeing her beautiful mouth), but *she hates it.* She has her nose fixed and is happy.

I know some people will say that she would then find something else to be unhappy about. Maybe; not always. A person who will *always* find something wrong is in need of psychiatric help, and a reputable plastic surgeon can spot that. He'd probably refuse to do the operation. Why should he go through the rigamarole? If the patient has psychological problems, no results will be satisfying. A *reputable* doctor will ask what the patient is really looking for and discuss whether plastic surgery is really the answer.

Even then, there is a tendency in patients not to be satisfied after the operation. Except in very special circumstances, a plastic surgeon won't do anything without cash down first. Otherwise the patient wakes up and, if he or she doesn't look like Paul Newman or Jacqueline Bisset, is ready to sue. The cash in advance shows you're serious and ready to take the risks.

There's more secrecy involved in cosmetics operations than in any other kind. I know many women who have undergone plastic surgery; I don't know whether a single one of them would broadcast the news. Though women are less touchy about the subject than they were ten years ago, you don't see much comparing notes on nose jobs or eye lifts either.

But plastic surgery is becoming more common as more young doctors enter the field. Their main job is restructuring faces and bodies of accident or war victims so they can return to normal life. Plastic surgery also corrects birth defects. But the patient who seeks plastic surgery in order to be more attractive isn't considered that frivolous anymore. A legitimate need is recognized. Psychiatrists will recommend plastic surgery when emotional problems arise from physical disfigurements that can be put right. Magazines and books are telling people more and more about the subject, bringing it out of secrecy into the open, describing the facts and figures of individual operations.

Plastic surgery is now accepted. That doesn't mean it's the way to instant beauty or instant youth. Yes, I'd go into a hospital and come out looking thirty if I could. But I'm not going to look thirty no matter what I do. There's no way a woman can regain her youth, and I don't think she should try. I can stand unashamed next to an eighteen-year-old when we're both in bikinis. And I know I don't have as good a body as she does. I can approximate but not compete with youth. A woman knows how old she is, and the surgeon's knife isn't going to delude her. She can look good, she can look better than she did, she can look fabulous, but she's *still* the same person at the same age.

I go to a plastic surgeon once a year to have him check my features and the elasticity of my skin. So far, he hasn't recommended surgery. When to have plastic surgery is not a question of age. It should be done the day before you need it, so there won't be a severe change in appearance to shock you and the people around you.

Once you decide to have plastic surgery, shop for a doctor with extreme care. Most of them are specialists, in noses, for instance, or eyes or breasts. Up to three consultations may be required before the surgery is done. If you can't afford it, don't have it done. If you're set on doing it, by all means get the best. Never go to a doctor of dubious reputation. He may charge less than others, but you're much better off with an unattractive nose than a mutilated one.

Certain beauty problems can be solved only by surgery. Stretch marks, for instance, from childbirth or obesity. Though oils, exercises, and massage might help avoid the marks in the first place, once they appear you can't get rid of them in any way other than surgery.

If you've let yourself deteriorate beyond a certain point, no beauty products can reverse the process. Several years ago I met a woman in Phoenix who was then in her mid-thirties. She was an outdoors-lover and did lots of horseback riding and tennis in the scorching Arizona sun. Her skin was almost black, it was so tanned and leathery. Her face was a mass of wrinkles from super-overexposure, and even the oil in her lank hair had been completely dried up. She looked twenty-five years older than she was.

Though I'd known her only a short time, I gave her hell for not taking care of herself. I told her that, unless she enjoyed looking like her own mother, she should go to a plastic surgeon. I gave her advice on skin care and make-up to use afterward. I knew there were possibilities of beauty in her: She was small and petite, with dainty features and a good figure.

I forgot all about the lady. One day in Palm Springs an enormously attractive stranger approached me, gave me a big hug, and thanked me for what I had done for her. I stepped back and told her she must have made a mistake. I didn't know the woman from Eve.

She told me her name and reminded me of our meeting in Phoenix. I couldn't believe my eyes. It was the same woman all right, but there was no way I could've recognized her.

She'd had her entire face lifted, including the upper and lower eyes. Surgery had removed the wrinkles and sagging skin. After the operation she'd stayed out of the sun and applied some of my make-up ideas. She had emphasized her eyes and lightened her mouth. Her long, lank hair now had a soft, feathery look. She was a different, and beautiful, woman.

She'd also had her face peeled. The texture of her skin had completely changed. **Peeling** is a cosmetic technique different from surgery. There are two kinds of peel, mild and strong. A mild acid peel gets your skin red and gives a superficial peel through mixtures of phenol; it's also used to burn off little warts.

The mild peel is sometimes nicknamed the "New York Peel," because models supposedly get it when they want to look really good for an assignment. They get it two or three days before shooting. Of course, the faster it heals, the less permanent are the results. But there's a tremendous romance about peeling, and some people believe that if you start out very young with a light peel, and go on doing it, you can keep from aging.

The stronger kind, the "real peel," uses acid and taping. It causes severe blistering and caking of the skin. The main disadvantage of deep peeling, outside of the pain, is the possible masklike result. It produces "pink" ladies, with skin like a baby's bottom that stops where the acid stopped. They can never be without make-up, for their own pigment will never come back. Light peeling can't accomplish that perfectly smooth look, but it does result in normal-looking skin without wrinkles. It makes bad acne scars tolerable, and minor scars attractive. Since it makes the pores contract, it can correct enlarged pores. It can't turn acned skin into peaches and cream, but no woman can—or should—expect it.

If you choose the deep peel, you will almost certainly undergo a lot of pain. You may be ill for days, unable to sleep or eat. In this case, you are trading extreme pain for a perfectly smooth skin. If you have a partial peel, in the mouth area, for instance, you may end up with a "monkey mouth": The skin around the mouth is pink, while the rest of your skin is darker.

For everything there's a price. A **face lift** costs a lot of money and will keep you out of circulation for a while. It may be painful, but if doesn't always have to be. A face lift, the most famous of all plastic surgery operations, can be done in a number of ways. It usually involves incision over half of the head; around the ears and above and behind the hairline. Excess skin is removed, the face is tightened, and wrinkles disappear. A newer type of face lift involves making an incision across the temple. Scars can later be covered by eyebrow pencil and wisps of hair brought forward. This type of lift is good for very wrinkly women, because it gets all the extra skin. But no two face lifts are exactly the same. A **neck lift** should always be done at the same time as a face lift—otherwise you have the phenomenon of a youthful face with an old, wrinkled neck.

People often wonder how long a face lift will last. It lasts forever. That is, the lift holds, but the aging process goes on. In a few years the person looks old again and may want another face lift. A few years later, another. And so on, until the skin has no elasticity left anymore and the face has become a mask.

Last year I gave my mother a face lift for Christmas. She loved it. She's very pleased with her appearance and doesn't bother about what other people think of her looks, though she takes secret joy when someone exclaims: "My God! You look younger than I've ever seen you before."

The doctor questioned my mother closely before the operation. She wasn't out to get another man; she loves my father. She wasn't trying to fool him by looking younger, just a little better. She didn't want to start a new life, and she wasn't out to please other people.

For my mother plastic surgery was not a *big* answer. She just looked in the mirror and wished she could look better. She wished she had taken better care of herself when she was younger, and felt that she had aged more than necessary.

She went through the ordeal, the swellings, bruises, stitches, without flinching. She bore up very well through the peels around her mouth, lips, and chin (a lift doesn't erase those lines). Now she's very happy with the way she looks. It was worth it—for her.

But in the case of a friend of mine, it wasn't. When her husband left her after a very long marriage, this woman was devastated. She decided on a face lift. But if she thought her appearance had made her husband leave, then she waited too long for surgery. She thought the operation would win him back, but he was already gone. If she were starting a new life, instead of trying to regain the old, maybe the face lift would have been helpful. But she can't get out of the past and doesn't know how to deal with the future. She's a sad person, and for her the surgery was a waste of time and money. She was completely unrealistic about the results of the operation.

For some women a face lift won't do much good even if they don't expect it to change their lives. Round, fat, chunky faces don't respond well to face lifts. An obese face with a short neck and chin won't show any difference. Overweight women should always lose weight before having a face lift, and sometimes the loss of weight will give a woman's face *all* the lift it needs.

I avoided plastic surgery many years ago, and I'm glad I did. When I was in the movies, first at Paramount and then at MGM, various producers and make-up people thought I should have my nose changed. They said I had a bump on it and I should have the bump removed. I did nothing about it, though, mainly because I was a coward.

Years later I studied photographs of myself and noticed that though I'm bad in profile, particularly my left profile, it has nothing to do with my nose. My jawline is indistinct and I have a singer's throat. My vocal muscle is prominent, far front and out on my neck. When this prominent thorax blends with my poor jawline, they fade away and draw attention to my nose. My nose itself is fine. I think it has character, and who wants a perfect nose anyway? My no-neck look doesn't need surgery—I just use darker make-up there and correct it.

Make-up can go far in concealing defects, but it can't hide a huge or hooked nose. The so-called **nose bob** is the most common and probably the most successful, long-lasting plastic-surgery operation. It can almost always be done in a surgeon's office. Except for black eyes, swelling, and bruises that fade away in two weeks, there's no aftereffect.

Bags and pads around the eyes *can* be concealed by make-up, but only up to a point. When the bags get really bad, or when the upper lids really drop, only surgery will help. For **under-eye surgery,** an incision is made at the base of the lashes. The fat cells are removed, along with a tiny bit of muscle and sometimes (but not always) skin. The fat won't grow back and no new bag will form. Removing that tiny bit of muscle means it'll take time for the skin to contract, but once it does it will be very, very smooth. Women with bulging or hyperthyroid eyes shouldn't have the lower lids done, or they will end up with an extremely pop-eyed look.

On the upper lid, the incision is made right in the crease, so it's invisible. Even before it heals, the scar is camouflaged by make-up.

Crow's-feet can't be handled by surgery, because the scar will always be visible. Peeling is the best solution there.

Chin surgery is rather tricky. To build up the chin, an incision is made through the mouth and an inflatable implant placed there (formerly it was foam). There's a 90 percent success rate, but problems can occur in the mouth.

In body surgery, the best-known is **breast surgery,** increasing (augmentation) or lessening (reduction) them. Small breasts can be made to look larger through padding. But for the no-bra look or the feel test, padding won't work. At one time silicone was injected into the breast to increase its size, but it "traveled" and was tumorous. Now no reputable surgeon will inject silicone in the breasts. In fact, the only place for injected silicone is in an operated nose.

To increase breast size, implants are used. They can be silicone jelly bags, some other synthetic, inflatable, or salt-water implants. Although the inflatable implants give a natural breast contour, their danger is that they can deflate. Salt water is the softest implant possible. (No, you don't hear the sea.) The breasts won't collapse, and they won't harden. They jiggle. The problem with implants has been that they must be softer than the normal breast going in, since an implant felt through the skin is harder than an implant felt on its own. Also, firm implants tend to get firmer after a few years.

A woman has to be realistic about increasing her breast size. She can't go from a double A to a D. She can, though, go from a thirty-inch bustline to a thirty-three or thirty-four. And no one should have to go through the emotional stress of being flat-chested or looking like a boy. If she likes the look, fine. If it disturbs her or makes her insecure, she should consider an implant.

Breast reduction is slightly more complicated. It's almost impossible to go through that operation without having visible scars.

When the breast is reduced, the nipple is moved. Formerly it was moved up, and some nipples were inadvertently obscured. Now it's moved sideways, and the incision is made on the outside, so women can have cleavage to the navel. The scar is covered by the arm. After breast reduction, breast feeding is impossible. So is nipple erection. Another example of the trade system.

Other body surgery inevitably leaves scars. It's sometimes done on women who would do better to diet, not undergo surgery. Thigh, buttock, and abdominal reduction leave long, linear scars. You can look normal in clothing, but you can't pass the bikini test. Body surgery often betrays a lazy patient; proper diet and exercise should do the trick. If those won't do it, there's a question of priorities: What's easier to live with, the unsightly scar or the unsightly bulge?

If you've decided to enter the exchange system and have plastic surgery, then choose your doctor with care. It's important to find a specialist in the particular operation you want to have. The price varies from doctor to doctor and from place to place. Usually, plastic surgeons charge what the traffic will bear, and there are no set costs. The initial consultation may be anywhere from fifty to a hundred dollars in New York or Los Angeles, where most of the best doctors are. The question then arises: Have the operation done in the doctor's office or in the hospital? The doctor's office is always cheaper. In a hospital, a face lift might cost five thousand dollars, including room fee, nursing care, laboratory, and the rest. The same operation runs between two thousand and twenty-five hundred dollars in a doctor's office. If you have a private nurse for twenty-four to forty-eight hours after that, you'll still come out ahead. But some patients, because of their life styles, require hospitalization. Usually, the doctor and patient together decide which is the best method for a patient.

Though prices will vary, here is a rough average of what the most-common operations currently cost in the Los Angeles and New York City areas:

NOSE SURGERY: L.A.: $850–$1500 (New York City: $1200–$2000)
EYE LIFTS (upper and lower): L.A.: $850–$950 (NYC: $1200–$2000)
FACE LIFTS (including neck and eyes): Starting at $2000
BREAST AUGMENTATION: L.A.: $1250 (NYC: $1500–$1800)

BREAST REDUCTION: L.A.: $1500 (NYC: $2100)

EAR RECONSTRUCTION: $700

CHIN: $300–$400 (but can include dental fees and go up to $1000)

THIGH AND BUTTOCK REDUCTION: $1000–$1500.

These prices are doctor's fees, for surgery and post-operative care only. They don't include hospital costs. Health insurance will cover plastic surgery only if the operation has improved the faculties of the patient—if an eye operation improves vision, for example, or a nose operation clears up breath obstruction.

While plastic surgery is expensive, the cost is even more than money. If you know what you want the operation for, and are realistic about its possible results, then go ahead. If you can look better and retain your individuality, you have nothing to lose with plastic surgery. But if you're relying on operations to improve you, and if each plastic-surgery operation only leads to another and then another, then you are indeed caught in the beauty trap. The search for perfection must be embarked on realistically. *No one* can reach perfection. If you work within the limits of your own assets and drawbacks, fine. But if you're always pursuing an impossible ideal, you're trapped.

13

The Beauty Trap—
and How to Avoid It

It isn't hard to fall into the beauty trap. All you need is basic insecurity, not enough sense of yourself. Then you're ready to be dictated to, ready to enter the treadmill, to be lied to, to believe in miracles. I've been through the beauty mill, I've been close to being trapped, and I survived. When I was married to Jerry an alarm would go off in my head every morning; I ran to put on my make-up before Jerry woke up. I was sure he would be horrified to see me *au naturel*. Now I do the reverse. The sooner I can let a man see me with no make-up on, the better. He can see what I really look like. If he doesn't like it, I no longer care to see him. I'm certainly not going to spend the rest of my life jumping up at four in the morning to make up for *anyone*.

At that time I measured myself solely in the reflection of others. That unsureness is the straight path to the beauty trap. It means becoming self-centered and not accepting anything less than perfection. It means investing in every wrinkle-removing cream on the market. It means going to the beauty parlor every day, or two, three times a week. It means spending many hours every day on narcissistic activities, visiting beauty spas, going regularly to plastic surgeons, trying all the fad diets and rejuvenating pills, following every new trend, and, in general, making beauty a fetish.

Any woman who spends more than ten or twelve hours a week on her appearance is perilously close to the beauty trap. At the opposite extreme, the woman who spends less than half an hour a day (and I include grooming activities) should consider taking better care of herself. To spend some time and thought on appearance is not entering the trap; it's part of asserting yourself. Two hours a day for beauty means trouble. One hour is fine. There can be exceptions. Once in a while I give myself a *self-improvement day*. Then I do my hair, my nails, give myself a pedicure, and generally pamper myself. It's fun and breaks the usual day-to-day routine. It can be a private time, to sort out your feelings and get your head together. If it's done too often, you enter the downhill treadmill of narcissism.

You don't have to be rich to fall into the beauty trap, but it helps. The very rich can afford to indulge themselves, in money and time, and go to beauty ranches. Not all beauty farms are filled with the rich, though; there are some for less affluent people who're also seeking to quench their thirst at the fountain of youth. And youth injections are available to anyone—unsubstantiated promises of beauty.

There is no way to attain perfection. God knows many have tried, but so far as I'm aware, no one has made herself perfect. I haven't. My entire life's work used to consist of trying to build up enough "yes" votes from everybody else to cancel all the "no" votes I've had going inside myself. If I could please everybody, that made me terrific, right?

Of course not. All the "yes" votes in the world from the outside are meaningless! Sooner or later you look in the mirror and decide everybody's wrong. Then all the self-assurance goes down the drain. And if you're living in the reflection of others, what happens when that reflection changes? That happened to me in my husband's eyes, and I was devastated. It was my fault; I'd indulged in the All-American theme of identity, where you see yourself through others. It's the need to please; it's self-defeating and a terrible loss, just wasted time.

We've been dictated to by beauty authorities for years and years. They give us conventional beauty, tell us how to look and how not to look; what is, and what isn't, acceptable. Ads set a standard of beauty, yet can be terribly misleading. But there *are* changes in the wind, and I'm hopeful the Beauty Mafia will be destroyed.

"Beauty Mafia" originated as a description of the beauty

business. It should be applied to those companies that try to limit a woman's appearance by time of day, time of year, indoors or outdoors, the kind of party she's going to, the kind of clothes she wears, and all that nonsense. But the only women who can be dictated to are those who lack self-confidence and have a need to be lied to.

I loved it when a famous beauty house announced false eyelashes were "out." That particular company didn't market false eyelashes in its line, and thought it could compete with the opposition by convincing women not to wear them at all. That's the Beauty Mafia at work.

It worked the other way, too. When false eyelashes were introduced, women of all ages were told they looked better with imitation lashes. The early models were inferior and made women actually look like they were wearing false lashes. Of course, millions of women have skimpy, uneven, or broken lashes, and false ones would correct them, right? So it became difficult for any woman to attend a party wearing only the lashes nature gave her. Even if they were full and long, they looked short and stumpy compared to the falsies. Then it depended on her sense of competition—how much did it bother her that every other lady in the room had her eyelashes beaten out by an inch?

Young girls nowadays are being more and more turned off by too much attention to beauty and appearance. They want to be judged on other merits, to be accepted first as human beings. That's fine, and I agree. The only catch is, if they're not happy about the way they look, they'll never feel comfortable about doing their own thing. I've watched Kathy and P.K. go through different and difficult stages of finding themselves, and they were at their best, their most secure, when they were satisfied and confident about their looks.

I don't think most girls today have abandoned beauty. They're just establishing new standards, looking in new directions. They are rejecting beauty products that are blatantly advertised as cure-alls for plain women. They're chary of the old establishment hokum. Ads that imply you'll get a man to love you only if you wear this lipstick or that eyeshadow turn them off.

Today's young women are too sophisticated for that. They reject the typical beauty ad with its sexual overtones. They suspect the ad that says this product "seems to" or "gives the appearance of." Such gimmicks are necessary to make the copy legal. You can't say in print that this cream removes wrinkles, because no such product exists. But the industry hopes women will skip the little clauses, see only "remove wrinkles," and rush out to buy the magic elixir.

Young women won't buy that. But they'll continue to depend on the beauty business for the products they do want. I don't see many of them whipping up their own treatments in their kitchens. They will also follow trends, but only to a point.

For more than fifty years Paris designers dictated everything a woman wore. And every woman, within her means, responded. We didn't have the self-confidence to rebel. Then we had the problem of trends changing so quickly and to such extremes that a woman's wardrobe was wiped out after a single year. Not many of us could afford to throw away an entire wardrobe and buy a new one. So now we have compromise. The trend is followed, but in combination. Pants tonight, skirt tomorrow, long dress tomorrow night. Each woman does her own thing, although she may try to stay within the general fashion dictates.

That's the best way. There are some women who reject beauty and fashion entirely. Some feminists believe a woman should wear no make-up at all, or pay no attention to her hair or figure. Fine. I never said a woman *has* to be beautiful. It isn't compulsory. I'll certainly agree that it's not harmful to your health to go without make-up or have your hair hang limp.

But maybe this extreme is just the flip side of the beauty trap. Some people depend on ugliness or plainness as a crutch. It advertises the negative feelings you have about yourself and forces people to react to them. If you run from all beauty products as though they were rat poison, or if you rush to buy out everything on the market as though you were an addict afraid the supply might run out, you're *both* caught in the same boat (or trap). You're showing your lack of self-confidence. You're assuming that what goes or doesn't go on your face is the most important thing in the world.

Most people feel better about themselves when they believe they look good. This doesn't mean competing with others. It means improving *yourself*, doing what you can to make *you* look better. Beauty isn't a commodity to be traded on the market. There should be no competition, because we all have our individuality.

What is beautiful to one person may not be to another; beauty is a changing concept.

When I was doing *The Polly Bergen Show* in 1957 and 1958, people said I was beautiful. Looking at photographs from those shows today, I appear outrageous. I'm wearing an "in" hairdo for the time, my make-up is modish, my mouth perfectly shaped. I am "beautiful" in those pictures by fifties standards, ridiculous now.

Beauty is as shifting as our lives. Pursuing beauty for the right reasons is healthy. Some women stop caring how they look after they get married, figuring they've now got their man and don't have to do anything more about it. But a woman should want to please herself. And it stands to reason that if she likes her appearance and develops her self-confidence, her husband or man will be more pleased too.

Many women are afraid of failure. They've lived so long with "I'm a great mother" or "I'm a fantastic housekeeper" or "My sister is the pretty one" that they've either forgotten, or never developed, pride in themselves as *individuals*. They feel safe in their old roles or hangups. Often they need some one or some thing—or the lack of someone, even—to make them want to change.

Often that thing is very painful. A woman is shaken to her senses when her husband leaves her. Or when her children ask why she isn't as pretty as other mothers. Then something's got to happen. And probably the best person a woman can turn to is her hairdresser.

Once started, a woman should experiment until she finds her own style, as I've counseled throughout this book. She should keep away from the reflection in other people's eyes and look in the mirror instead. No matter how much a man says he likes her thighs or breasts, she should look at them herself; she should look at *all of herself*, and make sure she likes, or at least accepts, what she sees.

Forget about other women. You'll never be like them or look like them. A Woman, with a capital W, is one who has put it all together, inside and out. She's beautiful to look at and beautiful to be with, because she is fulfilled. She's a Whole Woman.

It took me most of my life to learn this. I was so busy performing, publicly and privately, that I didn't establish my true self.

I didn't think about pleasing myself; my happiness was dependent on pleasing others. I haven't completely conquered that, and there are still contradictions in myself. If I'm interested in a man, I try to be what he wants me to be. I'm working for my own happiness—I want him to like me.

I said before that I am in the process of metamorphosis. I haven't shed all my old skin yet; perhaps I never will, not completely. But I am through with performing, in all senses. I'm honest with myself. And I'm working on it.

14

Who Says a Woman Can't Be President?

Were it not for Jimmy Stewart, a movie script, and grand-motherhood, I might still be singing and acting. Instead, the three elements combined to give me the most devastating blow I ever had as a performer. I was literally shocked out of the acting profession and into the beauty business.

I was thirty-three years old and had just completed *The Care-takers*—the movie I liked best of all I did—when I was offered a role co-starring with Jimmy Stewart in *Mr. Hobbs Takes A Vacation*, playing his wife. I knew it would be advantageous for me to accept the part. Jimmy was then at the height of his popularity.

I read the script. The part called for a woman with grown-up children who had children of their own. In other words, I was being asked to play a *grandmother*. At age thirty-three!

If you don't think that was a first-magnitude earthquake to my sense of personal identity, then you don't know actresses. I took a nosedive that is hardly believable. It was the most overwhelming psychological downer I have experienced, before or since. How *could* the producers conceive of me playing a grand-mother? I became terribly hung up about it. When I put the script aside, I looked at myself in a magnifying mirror for more than an hour.

Those tiny lines I'd always managed to overlook now became the Grand Canyon. Until then I hadn't really paid very much attention to my face—maybe because I was nearsighted. I panicked.

I ran right out and bought every beauty treatment and cosmetic I could lay my hands on. I bought some so-called magic cream that sold for seventy-five dollars, the goop that only neurotic jet-setters buy. I invested in the thirty-five-cent creams advertised on television, guaranteeing to you that three days after application a Rolls-Royce will stop by your door to deliver Prince Charming. At the end of three days, not even the paper boy stopped.

I went through every product on the market. I kept kidding myself some miracle would happen. Common sense finally told me there *is* no fountain of youth. So I thought that if I put something on my face in the morning under my make-up, it would keep my skin moist all day. I also thought it would be a good idea to put something on at night, for the same reason. But I wasn't satisfied with any product on the market.

And that dissatisfaction was the seed that eventually sprouted Oil of the Turtle, forerunner of The Polly Bergen Company.

One day I was playing cards with some girlfriends. A towel was wrapped around my head, and I wore some heavy, greasy stuff on my face. I thought that if a cream looked greasy, it really had to be doing the job. Right? That's how much I knew about treatment at the beginning. Actually, the greasier a product is, the worse it is for your skin.

Anyway, the girls at the bridge table were teasing me that I might be ultra-glamorous Polly Bergen to everyone else; to them I was a complete slob. I didn't feel like telling them I'd turned down a grandmother role with Jimmy Stewart, or the horrors of having other grandma parts offered to me subsequently. I just said mournfully, "You are looking at a woman who suddenly became Margot in Shangri-La. I went from thirty-three to one hundred and forty overnight."

One of the girls who heard my tale of woe about searching for a good moisturizer suggested I visit a chemist friend of hers. She told me he experimented in formulas for cosmetics and skin products.

"C'mon," I said. "It's all a racket. None of those things work. The formulas all contain the same stuff anyway. It's junk, and I don't want any part of it."

A few days later she introduced me to the man and, junk or not, I explained my problem, thinking it was uncommon. It wasn't.

Most women tend to think they are the only ones in the universe with a particular beauty affliction. Mine was a super-sensitive, dry, thin, flaky skin.

I told the chemist I wanted something to put on in the morning as a moisturizer under make-up, and also to put on at night. He said he'd make up some formulas for me to test for a few weeks.

Over a six- or seven-month period I went through about seventeen formulas. I kept trying and testing, my own guinea pig. One would keep my skin moist till noon. Another lasted until 2 P.M. Finally—I think it was the seventeenth—I took home a mayonnaise jar full of a formula that was to fulfill all my requirements. It really was terrific! *Extraordinary!* My face remained moist and dewy all day. I'd put it on at night and wake up with a fresh, moist face. I couldn't believe it.

After wearing it for three or four weeks, I knew it was sensational. Girlfriends asked if I'd had my face lifted. That sounds like a cliché, but it really happened. Next thing I knew, I was giving the solution to my friends. After about a year I discovered my gift-giving was costing me about three hundred dollars a month.

By this time, I wasn't working at a career. I was staying at home with my three children and Freddie, becoming Mrs. Freddie Fields for the first time. I loved it. I loved playing with my children and finding out more about them, spending all kinds of time with them. I became involved in charities on a fuller scale. I became active in SHARE, a charity working for the mentally retarded; I was involved in the Dubnoff School for emotionally disturbed children, and executive vice-president of the Women's Guild. I was enjoying my life.

But I was still hung up with the age thing. I sat down with my friend and fellow bridge player June Jacobs and told her we'd discovered something better for the face than anything in stores—why didn't we go into a little business? June is married to a highly successful Hollywood writer and didn't have to work any more than I did. This could be a diversion, and June thought it would be fun.

Each of us provided fifteen hundred dollars, and we designed a package. June became Head of Quality Control and worked with the chemist to make sure the product came out the same every time. She also made the deliveries from her garage, which was the warehouse. I did Promoting and Advertising.

But before we could tell the waiting world about our product, we had to give it a name. The formula was a combination moisturizer, night treatment, and all-purpose base, doing a little bit of everything. I thought all such products had the same basic ingredients, but ours must have some special catalyst that made it work differently from the others. I phoned the chemist and asked if there was anything in our formula that set it apart.

He made a thorough check of his charts and tests. "Yes," he said, "there is something. This formula has turtle-oil base."

"You've got to be kidding." Turtle oil? It sounded bizarre.

He told me that in ancient times people used natural, existing oils and that Cleopatra, according to historians, had used turtle oil.

Well, that changed it a bit. If it was good enough for Cleopatra, it would be just fine for other women. But the sound of "Polly Bergen's Turtle Oil" wasn't that great; in fact, I hated it. I was fascinated by the turtle oil, but I didn't see why the Polly Bergen part had to come in. Then I thought of the old play *Voice of the Turtle,* and even though it was about turtle doves, it gave me the idea for Oil of the Turtle. It sounds a lot better to say Oil of the Turtle than Turtle Oil. Don't ask me why, but it does.

I designed the packaging and June got all the components of the package together. But there was a little problem. I had a slight eye reaction to the formula. My eyes tend to be allergic when I put oils, creams, and lotions on my face. They itch, water, and turn red. When I told the chemist, he said the liquid entered my eyes and I should try the formula as a foam, which disintegrates and penetrates rapidly. A foam was made from the formula, and the results were fantastic—no eye reaction.

None of us had any idea that no cosmetics firm had ever made a beauty treatment product in the form of foam. Ours was the first foam moisturizer on the market. If we'd listened to the experts, we'd never have tried it.

Ignorance truly was bliss. We ran ads in little throwaway newspapers in the Los Angeles area—you know, those little papers you find on your front lawn at odd hours of the day and don't know how they got there. I drew up little coupon ads announcing the fact that turtle oil went back to Cleopatra's time, and asking readers if they wanted to join ranks with the famous beauties of history, at $6.00 per bottle or container of pink foam. The response was immediate; we sold out our first batch within weeks.

It wasn't a big deal. Sometimes we'd get five letters a day. We were having fun, and we enjoyed watching the sales increase week by week. We did all the mailing and labeling in June's garage, typing out addresses and putting them on the mailing tubes. Then we'd have coffee and relax. The business occupied us for an hour or two a day. We weren't making a profit, but we weren't losing money either. Just breaking even and having a ball. It was more fun than playing bridge.

We had no idea the business would grow much bigger. I have a feeling that if I'd known what the future held, I'd have run like a thief.

But business must always expand. June and I decided to place an ad in *The Los Angeles Times.* It was a major step; more people read the *Times* in one day than all the throwaway papers in a hundred years. I designed and wrote the ad very carefully, submitted it, and waited for the Sunday edition. When I got it, I searched through all the ads, then searched again—not a sign of Oil of the Turtle. I called the advertising department. They informed me our ad was on the pet page. They'd seen my drawing of the turtle, hadn't bothered to read the copy, and thought we were selling live turtles.

I had my first lesson in advertising. When a newspaper does something like that, the advertiser can have them run it again, free of charge.

When the ad was rerun the response was overwhelming. Then we began receiving repeat orders. We set up a little file of our customers. When two months went by we sent out reminders that their supply was getting low and it was time to order more. It worked like a charm.

Other women were as enthusiastic about Oil of the Turtle as June and I. We felt bold enough to run a small ad in *Vogue,* then in *Harper's Bazaar.* Now orders came on a national basis instead of just from the Los Angeles area.

Many times we delivered the tubes to the airport ourselves, to make certain they reached our customers on time. We were losing about two dollars on every tube we sent East, but we didn't know that, and didn't care. We were now national.

But we remembered our local customers. June went to a few small stores in Beverly Hills to see that the product was put on display. It was being seen for the first time somewhere other than in an advertisement. A year and a half had passed since our mailing and coffee. A nice little business was perking along. We were earning a tidy little profit and were devoting more and more time to work.

I was through with show business, but I had a single booking I'd postponed about five times at Harrah's Club in Lake Tahoe. My agency thought I should appear on talk shows to promote what I was determined to make my last singing appearance. They booked me with Merv Griffin, Johnny Carson, and Mike Douglas. Just before I was to go to New York, where Johnny and Merv were based, I cancelled the engagement at Tahoe for the last time. But I thought it would still be fun to appear on the talk shows.

The first was Merv Griffin's. As always happens on those TV talk fests, Merv asked, "What are you doing these days?" In the past I'd been able to talk about a movie or television show or night-club appearance. I didn't know what to say. But then, in a light, bantering way, I told Merv the entire story of Oil of the Turtle. He was interested and asked how his viewers could get the product. I said they could write to me in California. And that was it. I didn't give my address or say how much it cost.

June was in charge of picking up the mail orders from the Beverly Hills post office when the avalanche hit. It was four or five days after the Griffin show and I was still in New York. June was accustomed to picking up ten or twenty letters containing orders. But on this day the clerks came from behind the counter with three large boxes. More than twenty-four hundred letters had arrived in six days!

A week later Johnny Carson's show went on the air, and we received another twenty-five hundred orders. They were sent to Polly's Oil, Hollywood, Turtles, California, and other zany addresses.

The amount of the checks ran from fifty cents to ten dollars. It took June and me a full year to straighten out those initial orders, with sending back some of the money, filling other orders, and such details. We borrowed one of Freddie's secretaries to help out. It was the first time we'd called on him for assistance, but it was not to be the last.

I had an unlisted telephone number, but that didn't stop calls coming through from all over the United States. Department stores were going crazy because women came to their beauty departments demanding some of that oil from turtles that Polly talked about on television. The store managers, of course, didn't know what in Cleopatra's name their customers were talking about. So they called me in Beverly Hills. My agency and the Screen Actor's Guild were besieged by retailers wanting to stock the product.

Swanson's in Kansas City was among the first stores to reach me. Bill Heaton, head of the store, telephoned saying he was in town and wanted to stop by the house. I told him I was busy. I only had a card game going with the girls, but I told him he could stop by if he wouldn't mind waiting. Then in he came, president of that big department store, and sat in my living room while June and I and the other two girls continued playing. During a short coffee break we talked. I asked him what he wanted.

"Sorry to keep you waiting. I apologize. What can I do for you?"

He was generous. "That's all right," he said. "I'd like to carry your product."

"It's not in stores. We don't have facilities for wholesale marketing."

"That's OK," said the agreeable Mr. Heaton. "Just send me a gross."

That took a while to figure out, even though I'd been great in high-school math. It was the first time since then that I'd heard the term "gross" as anything other than the word that comes after reading "Motion-Picture Box-Office" reports.

Then it hit. My God, that was one hundred and forty-four tubes! We hadn't been selling that many in a week, except for the television deluge. I said it was a deal, and Swanson's was one of the first stores out of Los Angeles we went into.

When Freddie saw the new dimensions of our business, he told us there was an enormous potential for our product, and that we could make a great deal of money by getting out of the mail-order business and into the big retail-marketing business. June, who was the brighter of us two, said she was against it. Being somewhat slower, I said it was great. I saw expansion and growth ahead, not envisioning the work that would be involved.

Freddie, like me, is a diver-inner. You make the decision, then go full speed ahead. He said, "Sure. Why not?"

At that moment the business changed in concept. What had started out as a lark for us and our friends became a real enterprise, although I still thought it would be a barrel of fun. June was still a partner, but from then on things were different. Freddie and I provided the capital for the company, investing a considerable amount of money.

Oil of the Turtle now was a commitment. I began to seriously study and learn about the business I was in. I read as much material on the subject as possible, talked to everyone who would listen to me.

Van Vennari, cosmetics buyer for the I. Magnin chain, was a tremendous help. I just walked into her office, told her I was going into the cosmetics business and wanted to learn everything I could. (I realize now of course it didn't hurt to be Polly Bergen.) Van taught me the foundations of what the business was all about: products, sales, promotion, research. I began learning such terms as "thirty days EOM" (end of month), "FOB" (freight on board), and other foreign-sounding jargon.

Mike Meisler, a buyer in the Saks Fifth Avenue chain, was a great help. He told me that my packaging needed changing. My tubes were packed with a wrap-around label in pink. It was a gold-foil-and-pink paper, and not terribly expensive. Fine for mail order, he said, but it would have to be improved if it was going to compete visually with other products.

I took crash courses in dermatology from Dr. Alfred Lerner and Dr. Max Wolfe, learning basic facts about the skin: structure, pores, capillaries and the rest. And I tested every consumer product in every major cosmetics line to find out who was doing what. I was determined to discover who I was going to sell my product to, prices, ingredients, and how my product differed from the competition.

Freddie was the best help of all. He gave me office space, lent me secretaries and an office manager. Then I slowly, carefully, put together an organization.

I telephoned a great many of our original accounts, paid visits, and sold the product myself. Some—not many—called me. In those early days I didn't know one account from another once I was outside Los Angeles, Now York, and Chicago. I made some mistakes in selling to the "wrong" store in a town instead of the "right" ones.

"Wrong" and "right" depends on where you want to place your product. I had made up my mind it wasn't to be a mass-distributed line. I couldn't afford to choose bargain-basement outlets, because the product was too expensive. I had the kind of ego that needed the assurance of knowing my friends would want to use the product. So I was going to go first class—all the way!

I hired a man who helped redesign the product. The office manager worked out a projection for the first year's sales, predicting that we could sell one hundred thousand tubes to our original fifty accounts. That seemed a tremendous number, and I was quite frightened at the thought of it. But the office manager assured me we could sell that many.

I booked myself on every talk show across the country to promote the product. In forty-one days I covered thirty-eight cities and appeared in almost every single store that carried Oil of the Turtle. I was on literally hundreds of radio and television shows.

After the tour I was in shock. We sold out all one hundred thousand tubes in twenty-eight days!

We were left without any product to sell for six weeks. It took that long to get the tubes silk-screened, filled, and delivered. Only God knows how many sales we lost in that month and a half when women were surely going crazy trying to get their pretty hands on Oil of the Turtle.

On that first swing around the country I took a hairdresser, a secretary, and seventeen pieces of luggage. I was going from Florida to Minneapolis in the middle of February and needed a wardrobe for every extreme of weather. Then I'd spend only a day or day and a half in each city before moving on. I didn't have time to send anything to the cleaners. I started out young, fresh, happy, and bubbly. By the time I got to the last city I must have looked one hundred years old from lack of sleep and the enormous effort of making so many public appearances.

On tour I talked to women in all the stores and discovered they were searching for the same thing I had set out to find: a way *not* to spend hours at the make-up mirror. It sparked the idea of developing a new approach to skin care for active women on the go.

As I traveled from city to city I called June in Los Angeles and described the products I wanted her to start working on. Halfway through the tour I'd made up my mind I would move ahead from a single product to a line of beauty-treatment items.

A single product is often put on a shelf with the douche powder or hair spray, and I disliked that. No matter how good the product is, it can't do well sitting on the sundries shelf. I wanted to be out on display with Estée Lauder, Germaine Monteil, Charles of the Ritz and Elizabeth Arden. I wanted my product to be fantastic-looking, *not* hidden among the mouthwashes. Also, I had a feeling I could offer women something that was not available to them: a simple, straightforward, totally honest approach to skin care.

But before we could even start on that, I had to cancel the last stop of my tour, Minneapolis. I'd been testing on myself the results of our chemists' laboratory experiments. I wore only long sleeves in public appearances, because I had formula numbers on my skin in ink above the spot where I applied test samples of the latest experiment. When I'd take off my clothes at the end of a day, it was funny to see the numbers going up and down both arms. Then I tested night treatment while I slept.

Before I got to Minneapolis, one of the tests went awry. I put on an oil, to be used as night treatment, in Kansas City, and awoke to find my eyes were swollen. I did a local television show anyhow. The lights were hot and, combined with the oil, the result was disastrous. I was in terrible pain if I kept my eyes open. When I closed them, the weight of my lids was excruciating. A doctor told me I might have corneal burn, and said I should go straight home.

I didn't have to be told twice. It was the most hideous experience I ever had in my role as guinea pig, and the worst physical pain I have endured. The doctor gave me a mild pain-killer. I had a three-hour layover in Denver, then a long flight on to L.A.

I hated to cancel my appearance, because most store personnel thought a Hollywood actress would be temperamental and fail to show up for appointments. I had worked extra hard to overcome that assumption, and took pride in being on time, getting behind the counter and talking to customers. I still feel bad that I missed that last store.

But I'd never known such pain. By the time I boarded the plane in Denver I couldn't stop crying. Even light was unbearable. On the flight the crew asked the other passengers if it would be acceptable to turn off all the lights in the passenger cabin. I couldn't wear an eye patch because even that small degree of pressure was impossible.

Freddie was at the airport with a wheelchair and took me

straight to my eye doctor. It was two in the morning. I had severely burned both corneas. My eyes were bandaged for three days and nights. Fortunately, eyes heal faster than almost any other part of the body; in four days I was up and around again testing products. I'd learned the perils of being a beauty test pilot. But somebody has to do it. Why not the president of the company?

Now June and I began to apply my "experience" gained during the tour to reality. Together we conceived, tested, produced and delivered into the stores by September 1967 (six months after my tour) a line of treatment products. We had seven separate items: the original Oil of the Turtle Foam Moisturizer, Deep Cleansing Foam, Freshener, Night Concentrate, Deep Sea Bath Treatment, Deep Sea Soap, and Scrub, a deep-pore cleanser.

I hired an advertising agency, all women, who did a great job for us. As for the business itself, I was still doing all the purchasing. After learning the aerosol-tube business, I found myself learning the bottle business, the glass business, and the jar business for other Polly Bergen Company products. Then I got into various plastics, caps for jars, embossed labeling. It never ended.

Whenever I thought I knew all the answers, four thousand new questions cropped up. It was the most exciting and exhilarating time I'd experienced in the business world. Curiously, in its own way it was more of a thrill than *anything* I'd done in television or motion pictures. We were helping to make an infant business grow. I was fascinated by the fact that our product had become an absolute smash almost overnight. I believe we made four hundred thousand dollars the first year. Incredible.

After that we hired our own sales force and introduced a complete make-up line. Then a fragrance line, and a bath line. The continuing battle was competition. Neither June nor I had been prepared for the fierceness of cosmetics-company rivalries. I must say, in defense of performers, that there's less backbiting in show business than in the cosmetics business. More people are out to get you in the world of commerce than in the arts. Cosmetics is also one of the most expensive enterprises a business person can get into.

The Polly Bergen Company grew like Topsy. First it was one product, then seven, then twenty-three, thirty-five, and now eighty-two products. The investment was constant. Yet we still have one of the smallest lines in the business. Other cosmetics companies have eighty-two treatment items alone.

One reason for not overexpanding early in the game was economic. At one point Freddie and I had more than two million dollars of our own money invested in the company. It became too much for us to handle on our own. So we went public, issuing stock. That was my first major mistake as a fledgling business executive. The increased investment in new products required new supplies of money from the sale of stock. But almost as soon as we got the money, it was gone again, taken up by the growing line of beauty aids. So I made our first deal with a partner and sold part of the business to International Industries, the Pancake House company.

They were marvelous people but knew nothing about the cosmetics business or product distribution. They helped us with capital, but we needed more than money. We needed professional assistance. I didn't have the knowledge or time to run the company in a full capacity because I was traveling all over the country. Absentee executives just don't cut it.

Ultimately The Polly Bergen Company became a division of Fabergé—the details are much too technical but it was the happiest day of my life. I was with people in the cosmetics business who understood it and could give me the kind of management I needed. The firm was big business, with sound business heads leading it. Yet I in turn was able to give Fabergé a consumer-accepted line of prestige beauty-treatment and make-up products that would be an asset to their company. From the start it was a marvelous partnership, and still is.

Now I can specialize in testing new products. The Polly Bergen Company keeps me busy and happy moving from place to place. I'm much busier than I ever was as an actress, and business isn't as difficult for me emotionally.

The major drawback in being a businesswoman is that it's placed me in that terrible position of being a boss, a category I don't handle very well. I became overbearing and demanding. This trait carried over to my personal life with Freddie. I think it affected our marriage more than the traveling, since both Freddie and I have traveled all our lives, before and after we were married, individually and together.

We weren't conscious that our marriage was in trouble during the early years of the company. But the erosion had started. My preoccupation with the firm created a tremendous amount of guilt about my children. I felt I should spend more time with them. I still feel that way today, even though my kids are usually busy dashing off somewhere when I'm home.

I'm slowly overcoming the guilt feeling about them. They have lives of their own, particularly now that they're older. But also, the company makes it difficult for me to build a new personal life. It's become so time-consuming and demanding that there isn't time to find a man who'd have the patience each month to tolerate my being home three days and out of town working the other three weeks.

Could I give it all up for a man? A dangerous question, and I refuse to answer.

Curiously, when the company was in its deepest trouble and close to bankruptcy, I begged Freddie not to make a deal. My psychological response was to forget about the company, because I thought it had a lot to do with our breaking up. I thought if we'd let it go, our marriage would be saved.

Freddie's ego couldn't let the company go. Freddie is a winner, and he had as much pride in the company as I did. We *had* to make it work. Neither of us is accustomed to failure.

But my ego is not as big as Freddie's. Or maybe it's just as large but in a different respect. I'd rather have had my marriage than a career. Now I don't have the same options. Yet in many ways the business has saved my life. It fills the void left by my acting career and my broken marriage.

In honesty, I must say during most of my performing career I had a different public personality from my private one. Acting was an opportunity to show off a facet of myself that rarely came to the surface in daily living. Now I have a more evenly distributed personality.

The transition from show-business personality to beauty authority took a long time, and I'm still in the learning process. I discovered more women will stop me to chat about cosmetics than to say something about show business. They seem more self-confident and at ease now that they can think of me in terms other than performer. And I would a thousand times rather discuss the fascinating details of beauty than the dry bones of the theater.

When I entered the cosmetics business I was thirty-five years old, and a national survey showed my name could be identified by 95 percent of the people in the United States. I value that recognition factor. I hope never to abuse it. I use my public image to help sell my products. What is that image? I hope, open and down-to-earth. (Sometimes I'm *too* outspoken.)

But image and personal association alone don't make a successful business. Too many stars have made that discovery after lending their names—and only their names—to companies that ostensibly manufacture products supervised by them. That sells a product only the first time. Initially, I think, my products sold because my name was familiar. But I'm the cornerstone of my company.

I try to infuse a sense of integrity throughout my company. I don't believe cosmetics advertising should exploit women's insecurities. Perhaps I don't always succeed, but I try to tell women honestly that there are no miracles. I think, and say, that they should take care of themselves and that help is available. In a recent ad I said, "You can't stop aging, but you can slow it up a little."

The best way I can operate is by using the stuff myself and putting only those products in my line in which I fully believe. Then I can honestly talk to women about the qualities and explain the ingredients—and *results*—of my products, which really *do* work better for me than other lines. I don't want to imply that all my products are needed by everyone. Some, like my soap, are purely luxury items. My bath oil is a superb body treatment—but a lot of women don't need body treatment.

If something in my line doesn't seem to work as it once did, I drop it immediately. Fabergé doesn't want it in the line either. If I discover someone else is coming out with a new product that is better than mine, I strive to improve my own. There's a constant striving for improvement. It's competition, and Polly Bergen—the company *and* the woman—is right up there in the running. And I like myself better now. Maybe it will turn to love.

15

I'm Going to Love Myself Some Day

My childhood was speeded up, but my maturity was slowed down. Maybe one caused the other. I didn't have time to be a child; I was an imitation woman from the age of eleven, and I felt all my growing up had been done before I really became a woman. I'd been a performer since I was a little girl, and I relied on performing through most of my life.

I never exposed one inch of my inner self to anyone. I could never cry in front of anyone—except in frustration during the shooting of a movie. But I couldn't show tears or sickness to anyone I knew. My parents had taught me to maintain aplomb at all times. They taught me what they had been taught, and I learned that showing deep feelings is a sign of weakness. Performing also teaches you to suppress basic emotions. In my acting I could hide tension and pressure. My face conveyed serenity, although I could be boiling inside. That can raise hell with your stomach.

I knew about acting. As a woman I have faked sexual gratification many, many times. My friends tell me they have too. Women do far more sexual play-acting than men. A man performs or he doesn't. He either has an erection or not. Women have it easier. I'd been reared not to let anyone see me at a disadvantage.

I developed an image of competence—I was always in control, always capable, a woman of great strength. No one in the world knew who I really was, not even Freddie, not even me. I never allowed myself to think of what lay beneath the cool I'd built up

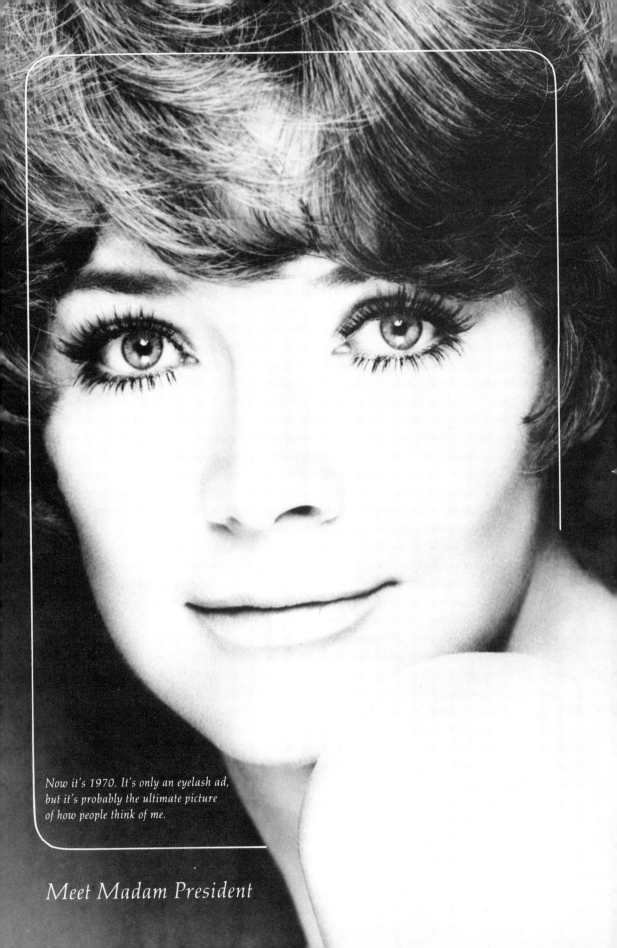

Now it's 1970. It's only an eyelash ad,
but it's probably the ultimate picture
of how people think of me.

Meet Madam President

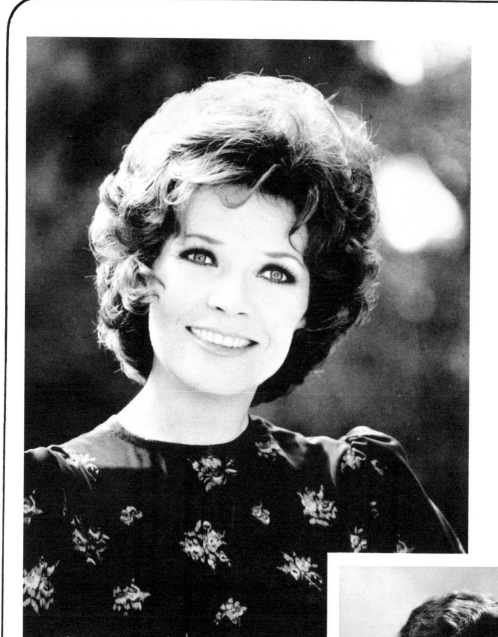

I keep running into the same (but wildly different) Polly Bergens light-years apart. Here I am at age 40 (above) and age 15 (right).

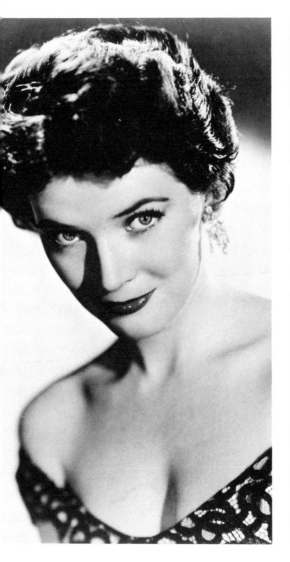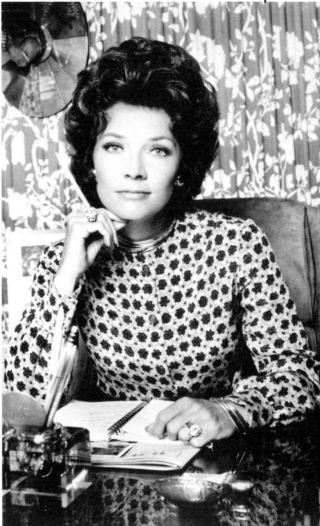

Ready for another case of how a woman can stop the clock? That's me at 20 (above, left) and at my desk at 42 (right). Of course, let's face it: a good photo retoucher can be a girl's best friend.

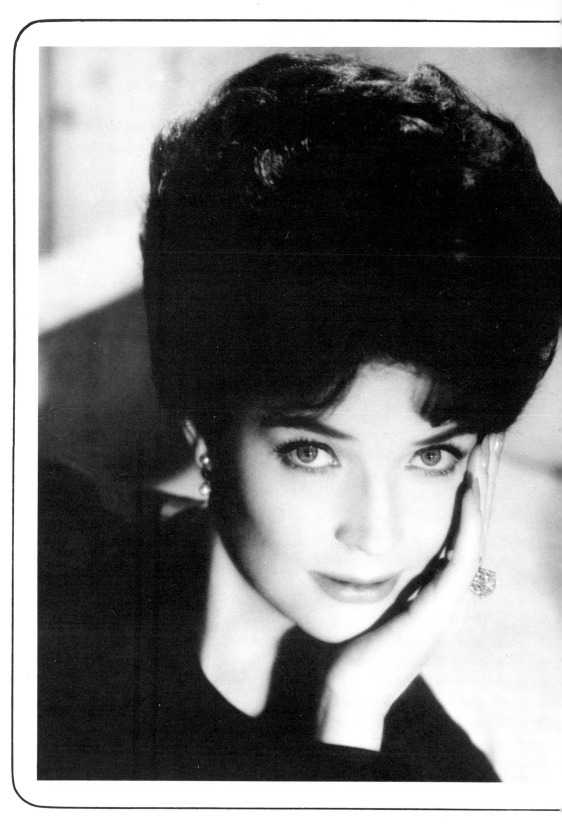

Still more and different looks. When the photo at right ran as an ad in Variety, *I was so cocky it didn't even mention my name.*

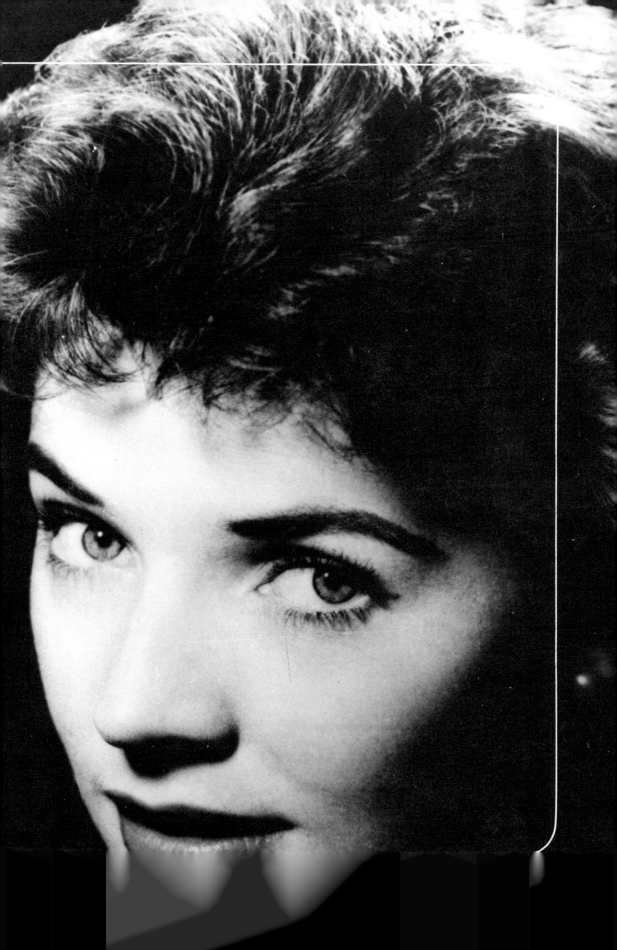

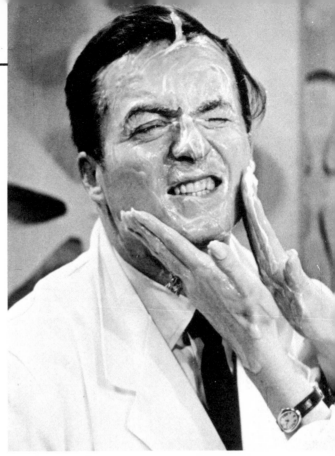

At 31, I was my most covered-up self (below). Nowadays, I know how to smear moisturizer on Mike Douglas on his show; manage the crowds at store promotions for my products; and ham it up at my presidential desk.

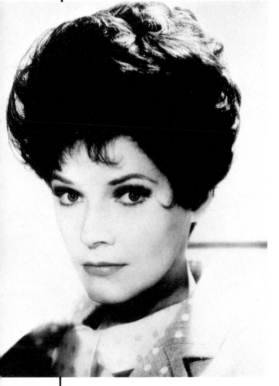

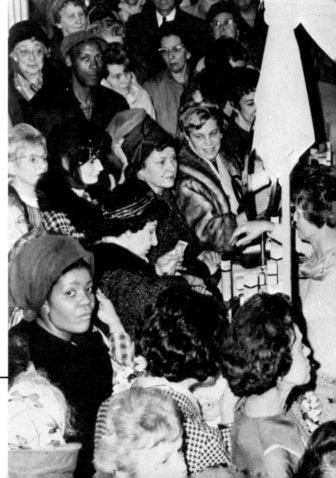

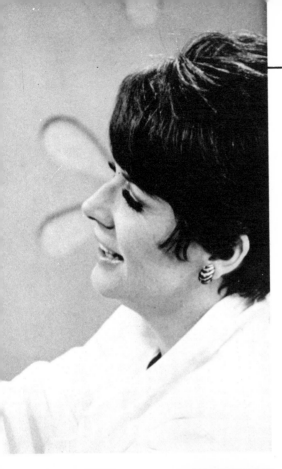

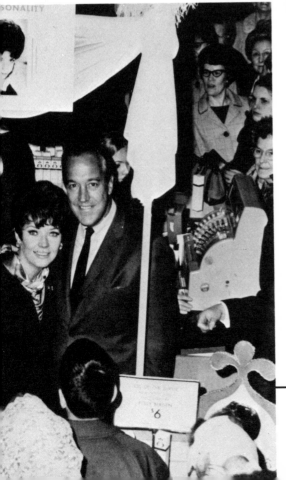

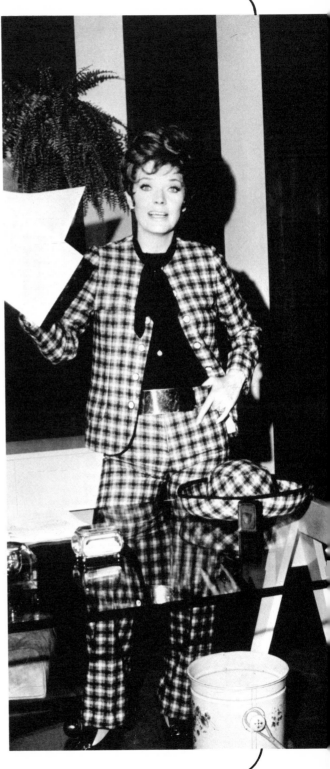

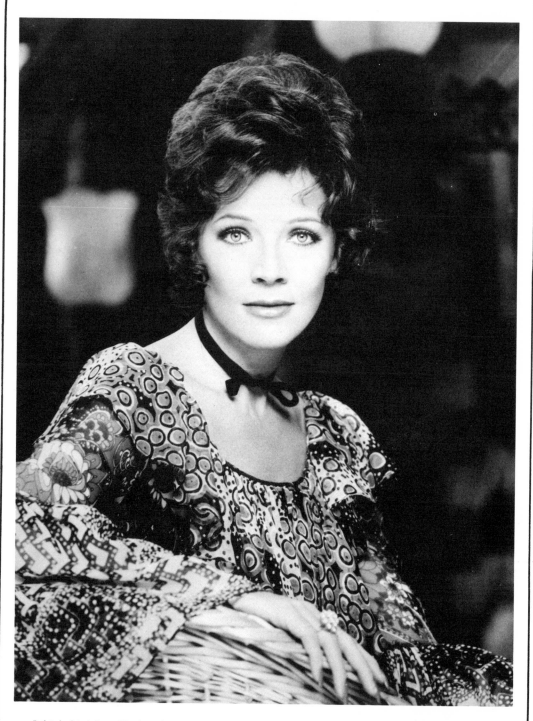

I think this is how I look to the people who are closest to me. I hope so. Because I think this is the real me that I'll get to love. Some day.

over a quarter of a century. Since my childhood I'd kept myself neat and clean, didn't laugh or cry too loudly, had my hair combed and my shoes polished. *But I didn't know myself at all.* I was insecure, convinced I was physically unattractive.

When I returned to Hollywood with Freddie and the children, I was offered many movie parts. One was the role that I mentioned earlier: an institutionalized insane woman. I wasn't under contract and didn't have to accept, but I fell in love with the script, and agreed to play in *The Caretakers.* Had I known then what the picture would do to me, I don't think I would have accepted.

The transference of fictional role to private life is an old Hollywood story. It's a switch on the Actor's Studio method, where you have to convince yourself you're a homicidal maniac before you can play the role with any verisimilitude. In Hollywood, or with television acting, the screen role can freak you out and make you into the sort of character you're portraying.

Kirk Douglas suffers from this chameleon tendency. "I'm a bastard to live with when I play a heavy," he told me once. "But I'm sweetness and light when I play the nice guy. I get too involved with my roles for the good of my private life."

Charlton Heston has played so many historical and Biblical characters, I'm surprised he doesn't run around Beverly Hills in a toga and sandals, with a laurel wreath on his head.

But instead of playing a lady or a beauty-contest winner, I picked a lunatic. Then I had the choice of playing it as a cliché or trying to break some new ground. I didn't want to fake it. It was my first opportunity since *The Helen Morgan Story* to give an outstanding performance.

My casting was certainly offbeat. The always-in-control-Polly was dealing with a woman who was thoroughly vulnerable. She was an open wound. To play her realistically, I had to seek out all the facets in myself that frightened me most, or that I was most ashamed of, and bring them out in the open to use.

I checked into the psychiatric ward of the California State Hospital at Camarillo for a few days, to study the women there. For the first time in my marriage to Freddie, I put something ahead of him and the family: my role as madwoman. I wasn't even aware of how Freddie and the children were reacting to me. Most of those weeks are blank; I don't remember how I behaved or my state of mind. The woman became an integral part of me. Or I became submerged in her. I don't know which, our identities became so confused in my mind. And I learned, in the course of the film, that the line between sanity and insanity is terribly narrow, and depends on emotional stability or the lack of it.

When I finished *The Caretakers* I was a basket case. I didn't know how to return to being the Polly Bergen I had always been. I wasn't able to sleep or to hold an intelligent conversation for more than a few minutes. All those fences I'd erected, the self-contained world I'd built for myself, crumbled. I couldn't function any more. I couldn't deal with my problems. Until then I couldn't understand why people were unable to cope, and I thought someone who couldn't solve the minor irritations of life was weak. All of a sudden I was that person.

I went into therapy. I had to. I began to make some changes in my life. I opened up and became vulnerable for the first time. Freddie was the one I opened up to—the first person and the first time. I exposed my weaknesses to him and he reassured me, telling me it was OK, telling me he still loved me.

The one thing I feared most in life—not belonging to anyone—disappeared. And, curiously, for the first time in my life I fell in love—with Freddie. I had loved him before in the limitations of what I *thought* was love. Now I could give of myself, and I gave myself to Freddie. I also became closer to my friends.

But then I withdrew. The type of therapy I was going through was too strong, it demanded too much of me too soon. So I went instead to Dr. X, a psychologist. He was bright and loved show-business personalities. Instead of meeting him on an honest basis, I performed. My defensive attitude was there, and I couldn't discuss my innermost problems. I acted the person I was "supposed" to be. Dr. X pointed out that I never lost my temper. He was right, and it's still hard for me to do. When I blow up, I literally, physically fall down. My knees buckle, and if I can't grab onto someone or something, down I go.

Since I couldn't stop performing for Dr. X, I finally left him, and then avoided analysis for several years. My life was glamorous; we entertained a lot and I was starting my company. I had a good life and seemed to be happy. But Freddie and I were losing our ability to communicate, and indifference was beginning to set in. I went to a marriage counselor, but Freddie wouldn't take part in the counseling, and she suggested I try group therapy.

I spent a year with the group. The main approach, at least in my group, was attack, attack, attack. I was at a disadvantage, since they all knew me from my work and I didn't know any of them. Here I was, super-self-critical to begin with, now beating myself up and allowing six other people to work me over verbally. The extra criticism was difficult to bear, but I went on with it, thinking it would strip my reluctance to be honest with people and with myself.

For the first time I learned about male weaknesses and insecurities. Both my father and Freddie seemed to have such strong egos that I assumed all men were as confident and able to take care of themselves. Now I saw the male without his armor, and I saw that he could be weak, and vulnerable, and frightened. It was a revelation.

I realized I had demanded *too* much of Freddie. In demanding only strength from him, I never allowed him to show me any weakness. It didn't occur to me that the possibility of weakness was there. I'd thought male weakness was bad, just as I'd thought female strength was unfeminine. I'd lived with absolutes, believing that men never cried and never showed emotion except for humor, sexual desire, and anger.

In living up to the picture I painted, Freddie must have been under enormous stress. Freddie had to be *my* strength, *my* guide, *my* father, husband, boyfriend, and *my* lover. I turned to him whenever I couldn't handle the children, depending on him to lay down the law and enforce it. He was *my* guide in *my* career. He had to be like a father so I could lean on him and pour out my problems. My expectations of him were too much, and I think now it's no wonder he finally gave up trying. I put on him the same sort of pressure a man puts on a woman when he treats her like a goddess, a beautiful daughter, a precious trinket. In a sense, though, Freddie also had his expectations of me. I was his madonna, and I'm not one and don't ever want to be.

When I realized Freddie and I were not going to make it as man and wife, I quit the group. I'd gone as far as possible with that sort of therapy. Only after my separation did I find Dr. Z, a psychologist who has opened doors of awareness for me. We have a harmonious relationship and complete accord. I think if I had gone to Dr. Z in the first place my marriage could have been saved, and a lot of the heartbreak avoided. I'm second-guessing, of course. But through this doctor my old actressy self has finally been cast aside.

When I came to him I said, "I know psychiatry doesn't have any magic wands. And I know you can't perform miracles."

"Wait a minute!" he said, stopping me. "You're making predictions and evaluations without knowing what it's really about. In fact, I *do* have a magic wand. And I *can* perform miracles. Well—at least I can give you tools that will allow you to function better, tools *you* can use."

He gave me those tools (or wands?), and as I write this book I'm still visiting Dr. Z. He's largely responsible for me being able to talk frankly about my life. Unlike most of the people I've known, he doesn't make judgments about me. And if I make a judgment, he pins me down and asks why. He helps me understand why I have certain feelings, attitudes, moods.

I now don't think it's a sign of weakness to get psychological or psychiatric help. If you need it, get it. I was very unreasonable thinking I could handle everything myself. That's like trying to cap your own teeth. It's no easier to get your own head straightened out than to work on your own molars. Peace of mind is the best beginning for everything, including beauty. Without a tranquil mind, an acceptance of yourself, it's impossible to feel well. *And if you're not feeling well, the odds against looking well are enormous.*

The change in me was reflected in different ways. I changed my style of dressing, wearing clothes that revealed my body more and going without underwear. I lost ten pounds. My new wardrobe helped change my attitude about myself, but the new wardrobe was a result of my digging into the self-approval hangup. I realized nobody else can make me bad or good or guilty or unattractive or unwanted. Only I can do that. If someone makes me think some way about myself, it's because I gave him that power. All I have to do is take it away. No one can make me feel unattractive anymore, because I tell myself, "I haven't given them that power."

But there are times when I don't like the way I act. When I'm in my role as president of a cosmetics company, some people see a driven, hard-boiled businesswoman in control of herself and her milieu. These people may think I'm a very aggressive woman, for I'm aware of the vibrations I give off in those circumstances. I don't like them. There's an aggressive, nasty, intimidating, killer kind of quality I have hidden in me which I'm trying to eliminate.

That particular Polly Bergen is unbeautiful and unpleasant. She comes out when I'm frightened, under pressure, or extremely nervous. The only way to stop her is if someone else says, "Hey, that's not you. You're frightened or you're nervous." My doctor does that. And I remember Freddie treating me as if I were a client when I flew off the handle. He was afraid of my reaction if he treated me honestly.

My performing still goes on. The forces of my life can't be changed overnight, but by being honest with myself, at least I can see what I'm doing and try to put an end to performing.

There are levels of performing, or role-playing, though. The danger comes when the role-playing is everything, when the act is all you've got. Certainly, everyone performs to some degree. We're different with strangers than we are with the family, and we're different with them than with friends. We adjust ourselves to public and private life. With a small group of close friends we're not the same as at a big, formal party wearing evening gowns. When a woman dates a man, she doesn't immediately expose him to her faults. So she puts on a performance, and so does he.

Usually I try to fit my date's preconceptions of me. I don't know if I'm actually performing at the beginnings of those relationships, because a variety of people exists within me. It's true of everyone. Sometimes I feel like a dependent girl or a sophisticate or a no-nonsense businesswoman. Then I just bring whatever it is to the foreground.

I keep tuning my personal radio until I get the wavelength to which a man responds best. Then I tune up the volume and that's the number I play. There are two sides to performing. One is in trying to please people, emphasizing some part of you, and it's fun. The other is destructive, a faking out. When I first meet a man I like, I show him sides of me that will make him interested. But as the relationship goes on, I show him the rest of myself. I've had some affairs since my marriage ended. None of them has been an end-of-the-world romance. But they have been honest relationships. After the first come-on (isn't that part of flirting?), I've been forthright about who I am and how I really look. I can take off my make-up—the party's over.

I've learned to flirt, to relax, to let a man approach me. I had built up a façade of protective armor which said: "Don't touch, I'm not available." I've been married a total of twenty-two years (five to Jerry, seventeen to Freddie), and most of my life was built around a husband (and children). My generation was taught that a woman's only goal in life is marriage and children, and that no decent woman goes to bed with a man she isn't married to. Now, for the first time, I'm facing the fact that marriage might not be the answer.

The happily-ever-after syndrome of marriage can be a fantasy, something to hope for, to dream of perhaps, but not to trust your life to. Relationships and their growth come from interpersonal understanding, not from a contract. I realize now that marriage can be almost a business transaction. Two people who trust each other make a business deal but never sign a contract. They trust each other enough to know the deal will work for as long as it's supposed to work, and they shake hands on it. Two people who don't trust each other will demand a contract.

I've learned too that a woman can't build her life on a man, or just for men. That sort of dependence can make a woman forget who she is. It can make her dissatisfied with herself.

My present goal is to be happy with me, to accept and fulfill myself. The effort can be very difficult. It can be depressing when you flunk a test you've set up for yourself. I still flunk communication with the children sometimes. I know it's a common problem and has to do with the generation gap. But I realize I can't handle the differences between them and myself until I'm first able to deal confidently with me. But I love them and it's worth the effort.

I'm determined to end my performing. I'm determined to be honest with myself. If I can accomplish these goals, I can accept myself as beautiful. And then—I'm going to love myself, some day.

Index

About the Author

Polly Bergen is president of The Polly Bergen Company, a subsidiary of Fabergé. She created the company in 1965. It produces a complete line of beauty products.

Before being a company executive, Miss Bergen was one of the most versatile performers in show business. She was a singer, dancer, and actress, on stage, screen, and television and on records. She is perhaps best remembered for her award-winning performance in *The Helen Morgan Story* and as a wacky panelist on *To Tell The Truth.*

She has long been regarded as an authority on fashion and beauty.